Hysterectomy - Past, Present and Future

Edited by Zouhair Odeh Amarin

Published in London, United Kingdom

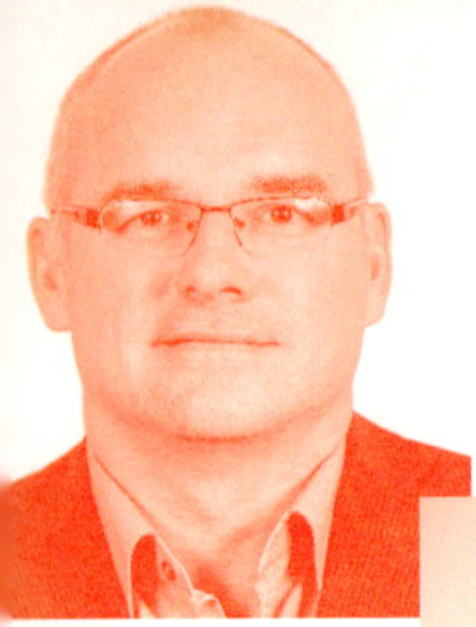
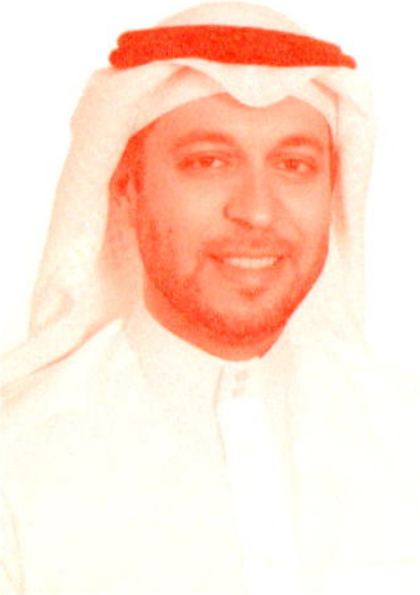
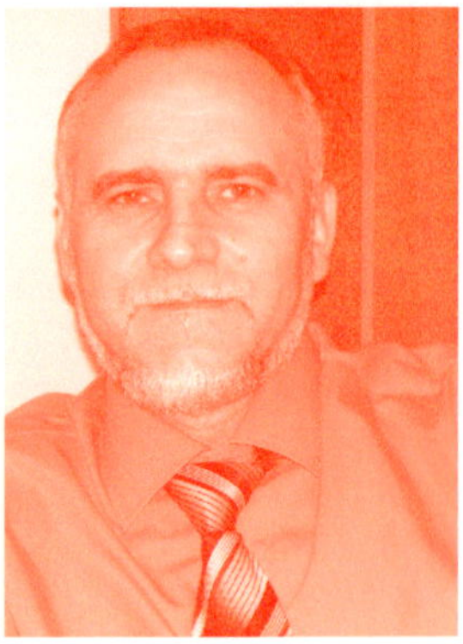
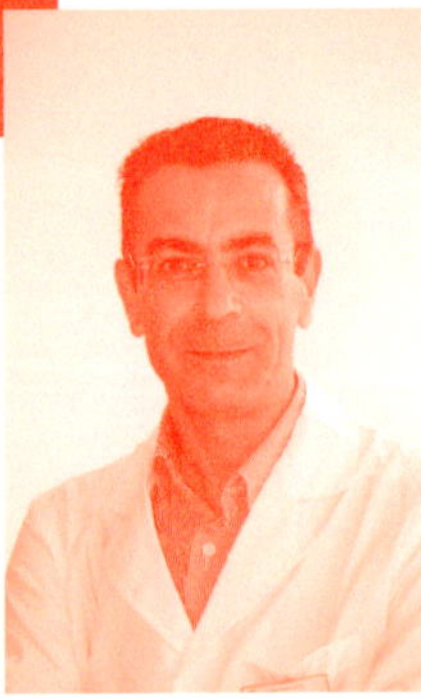
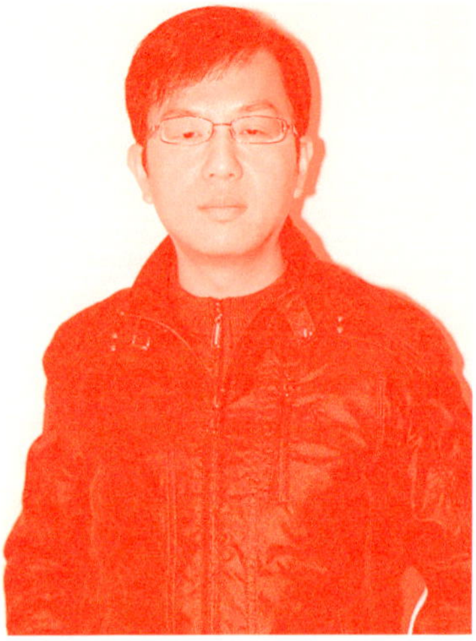
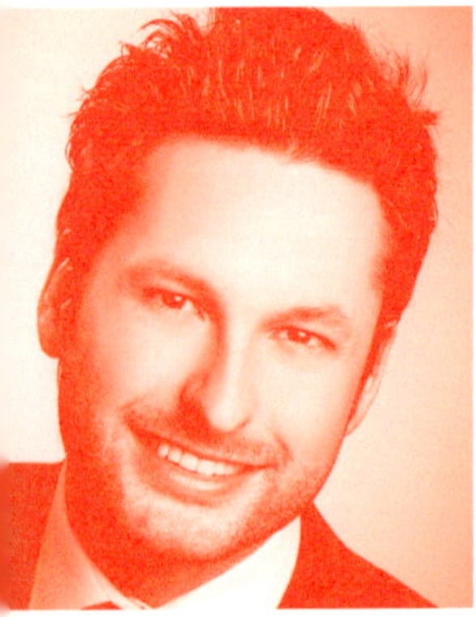
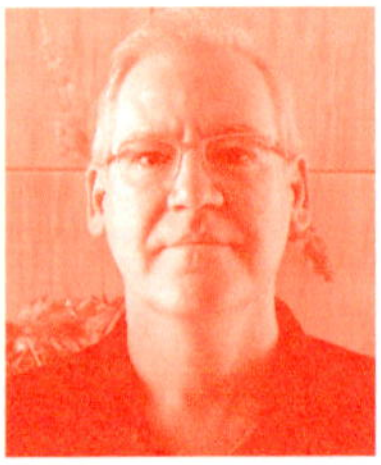

IntechOpen

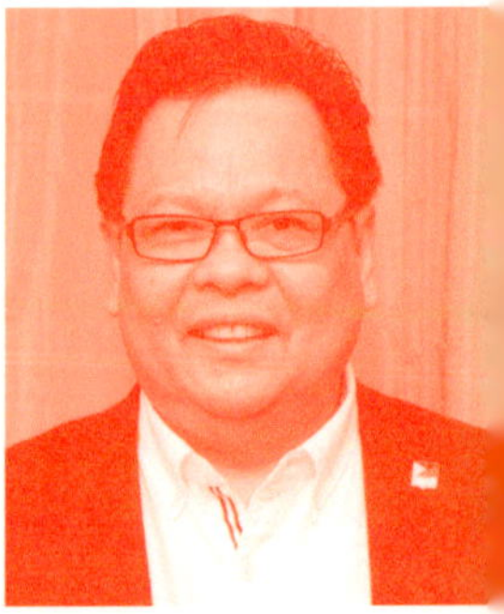
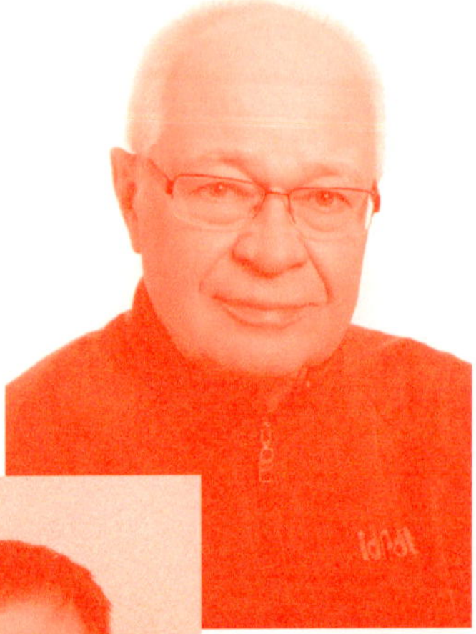
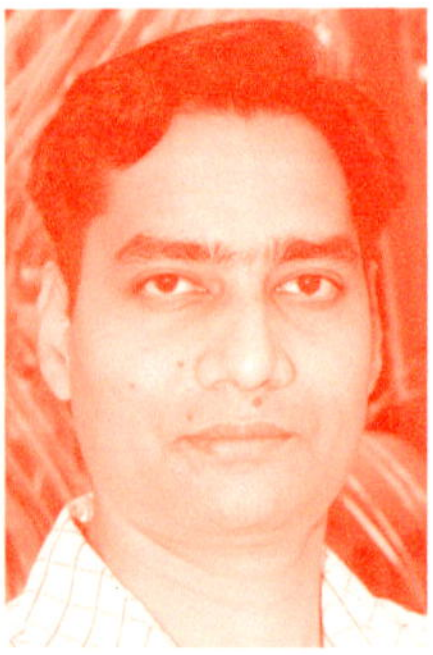
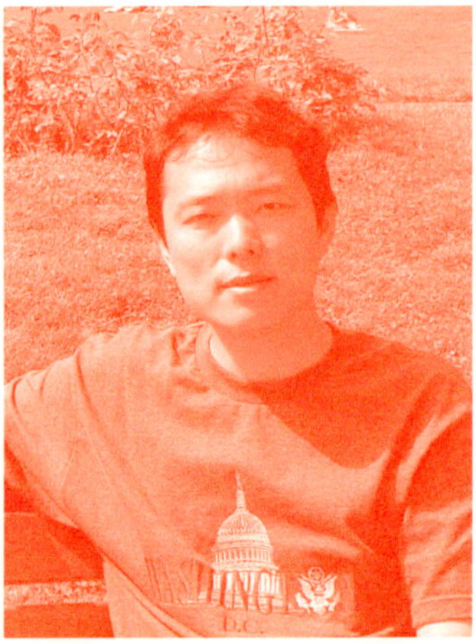
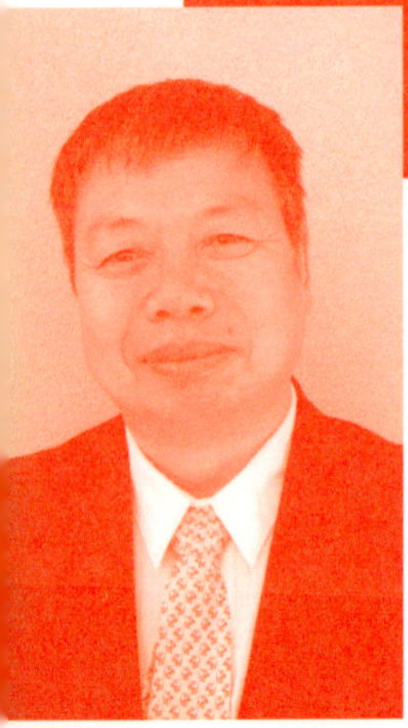
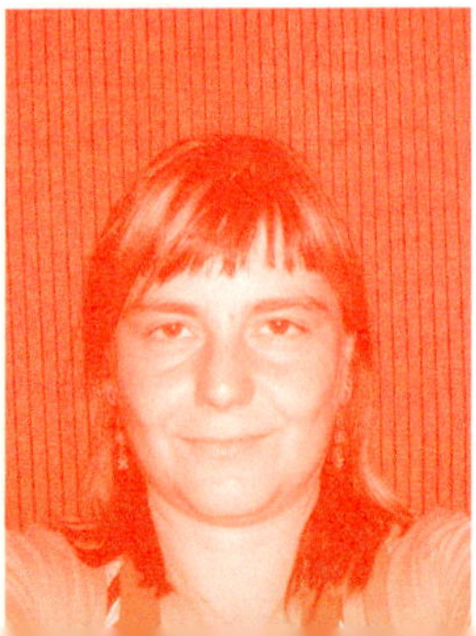

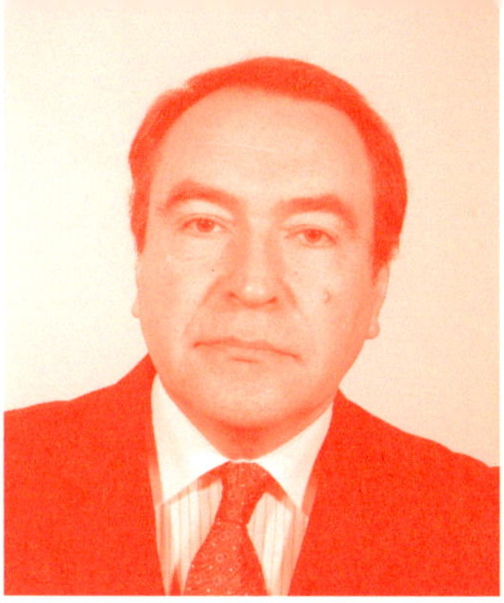

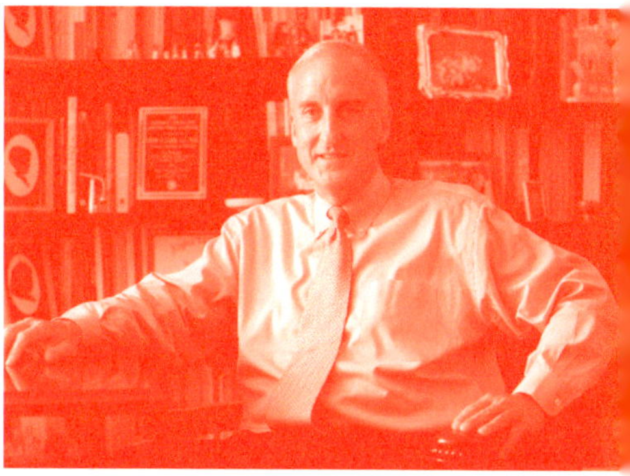

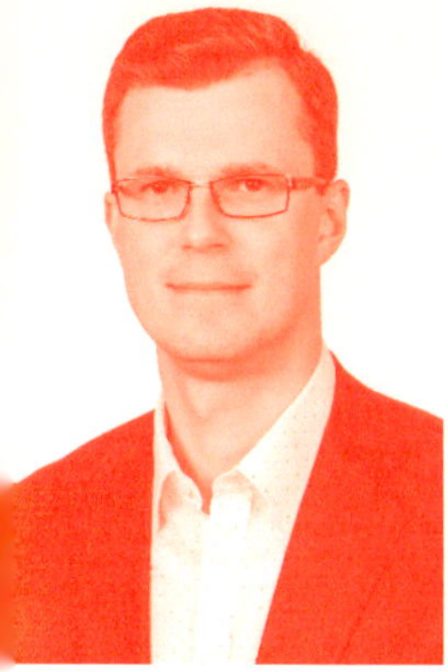

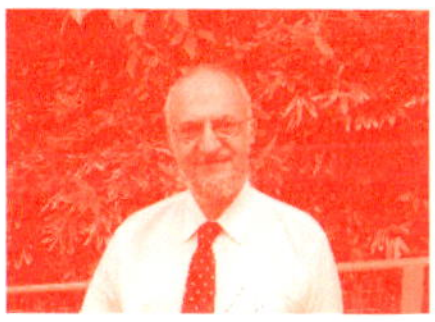

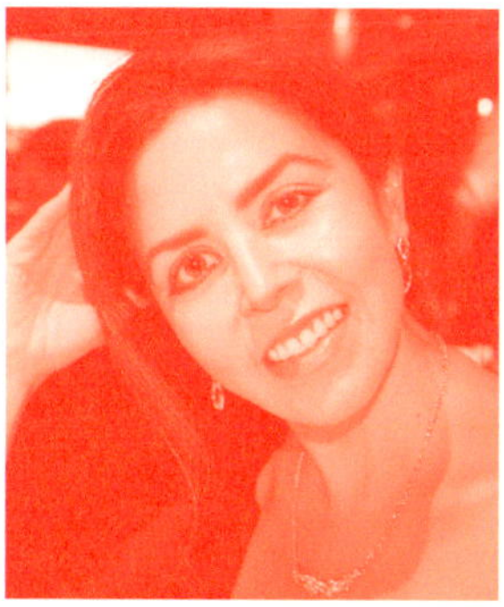

Supporting open minds since 2005

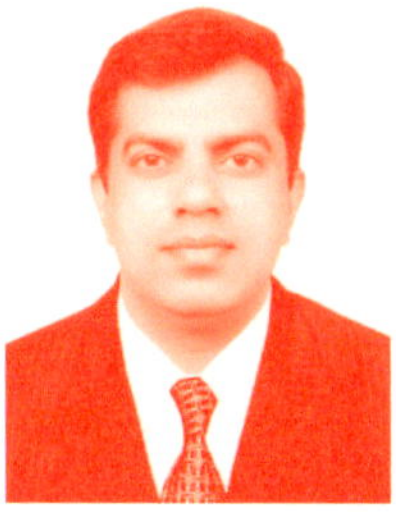

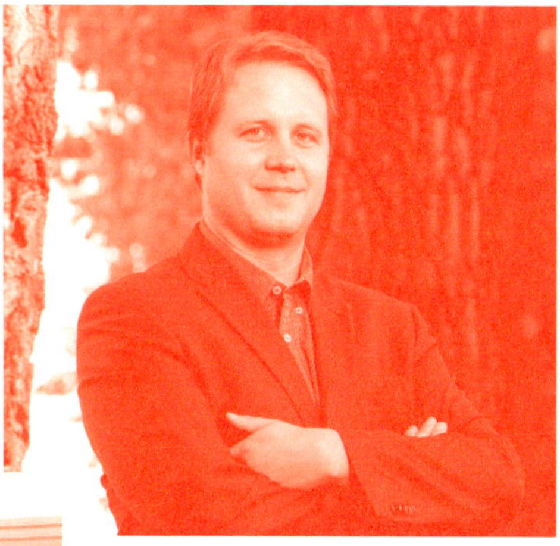

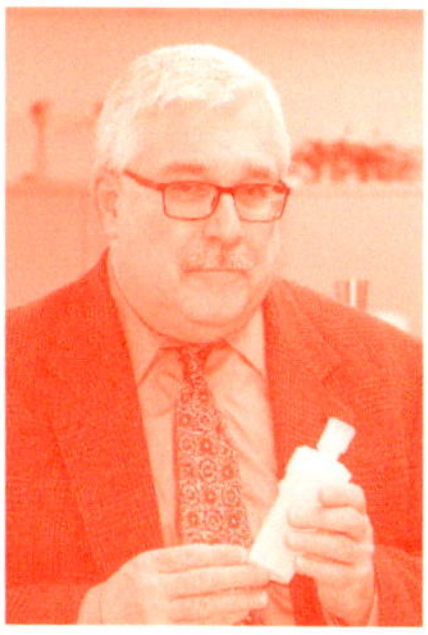

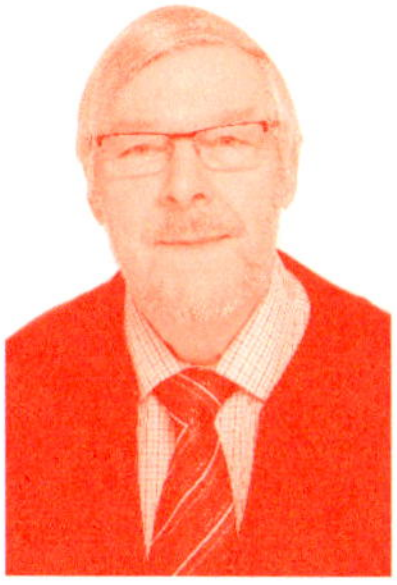

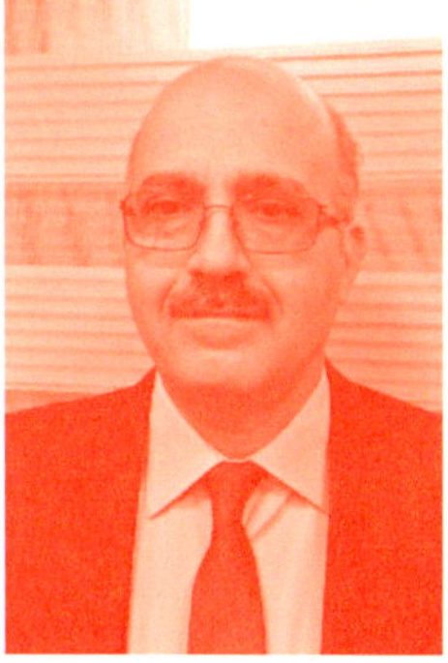

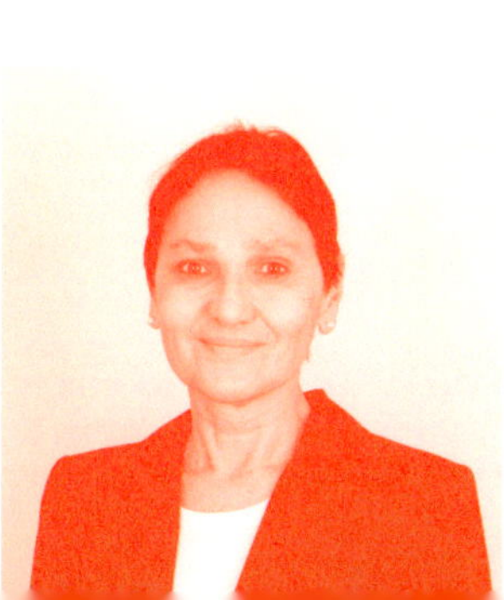

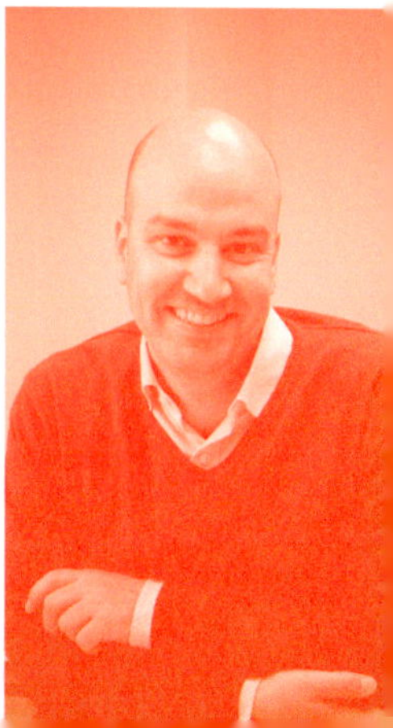

Hysterectomy - Past, Present and Future
http://dx.doi.org/10.5772/intechopen.95738
Edited by Zouhair Odeh Amarin

Contributors
Adriana Fulginiti, Martin Michalewski, Robert A. Graebe, Frank Borao, Michael L. Nimaroff, Catherine W. Chan, Masoud Azodi, Annemieke Wilcox, Merima Ruhotina, Shabnam Kashani, Johnstone Shabaya Shabaya Miheso, Eugen Ancuta, Radu Zamfir, Eduard Crauciuc, Gabriel Martinescu, Dumitru Sofroni, Larisa Sfroni, Lilian Gutu, Codrina Ancuta, Dragos Valentin Crauciuc, Petre Bratila, Amornrat Ratanasiri, Thawalsak Ratanasiri, Natakorn I. Tuporn, Somnuk Apiwantanagul, Thitima Nutravong, Thawalrat Ratanasiri, Zouhair O. Amarin

First published in London, United Kingdom, 2022 by IntechOpen
IntechOpen is the global imprint of INTECHOPEN LIMITED, registered in England and Wales, registration number: 11086078, 5 Princes Gate Court, London, SW7 2QJ, United Kingdom
Printed in Croatia

British Library Cataloguing-in-Publication Data
A catalogue record for this book is available from the British Library

Additional hard and PDF copies can be obtained from orders@intechopen.com

Hysterectomy - Past, Present and Future
Edited by Zouhair Odeh Amarin
p. cm.
Print ISBN 978-1-80355-060-2
Online ISBN 978-1-80355-061-9
eBook (PDF) ISBN 978-1-80355-062-6

For EU product safety concerns:
IN TECH d.o.o., Prolaz Marije Krucifikse Kozulić 3, 51000 Rijeka, Croatia, info@intechopen.com or visit our website at intechopen.com.

Meet the editor

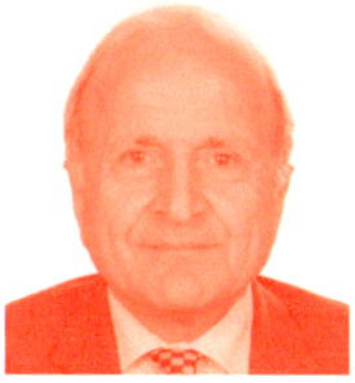

Zouhair Odeh Amarin is a Professor of Obstetrics and Gynaecology at the Jordan University of Science and Technology. Previously, he was a lecturer at the University of Glasgow, Scotland; senior lecturer at the University of Nottingham, United Kingdom; and dean of the Faculty of Medicine, Mutah University, Jordan. He is a fellow of the Royal College of Obstetricians and Gynaecologists and the Faculty of Public Health, London. He has a master's degree in Medical Science from the University of Glasgow, and a master's degree in Medical Education from Maastricht University, The Netherlands. Dr. Amarin is a pioneer in in-vitro fertility and was the first to develop microsurgical epididymis sperm aspiration for clinical use. He also discovered a surgical procedure for critical ovarian hyperstimulation syndrome. He is the author of numerous book chapters, editor of several books, and author of more than 120 journal papers. Dr. Amarin is also the recipient of eight awards.

Contents

Preface XI

Chapter 1 1
Hysterectomy: Past, Present and Future
by Zouhair Odeh Amarin

Chapter 2 9
From Open to Minimally Invasive: The Sacrocolpopexy
by Adriana Fulginiti, Frank Borao, Martin Michalewski and Robert A. Graebe

Chapter 3 27
Perspective Chapter: Total Vaginal Hysterectomy for Unprolapsed Uterus
by Petre Bratila

Chapter 4 55
Laparoscopic Hysterectomy in Morbidly Obese Patients
by Merima Ruhotina, Annemieke Wilcox, Shabnam Kashani and Masoud Azodi

Chapter 5 69
Bleeding after Hysterectomy: Recommendations and What to Expect
by Eugen Ancuța, Radu Zamfir, Gabriel Martinescu, Eduard Crauciuc, Dumitru Sofroni, Larisa Sofroni, Lilian Guțu, Codrina Ancuța and Dragoș Valentin Crauciuc

Chapter 6 85
Surgical Site Infection after Hysterectomy
by Catherine W. Chan and Michael L. Nimaroff

Chapter 7 95
Cases of Postpartum Hemorrhage and Hysterectomy in Thailand's Northern and Northeastern Provincial Hospitals
by Thawalsak Ratanasiri, Natakorn I. Tuporn, Somnuk Apiwantanagul, Thitima Nutrawong, Thawalrat Ratanasiri and Amornrat Ratanasiri

Chapter 8 107
Management of Vaginal Vault Prolapse after Hysterectomy
by Johnstone Shabaya Miheso

Preface

All aspects and techniques of hysterectomy are already well described in many publications, but to be adequately experienced, the surgeon needs extensive clinical operative practice. As such, this book discusses the techniques of hysterectomy, how to choose the appropriate method and potential complications of this surgical procedure. It also presents a brief history of hysterectomy and possible future directions in the field.

I would like to thank all the authors for their valuable contributions. I am also grateful to Author Service Manager Ms. Mia Vulovic and the commissioning editors at IntechOpen for their support and advice.

Zouhair Odeh Amarin
Jordan University of Science and Technology,
Irbid, Jordan

Chapter 1

Hysterectomy: Past, Present and Future

Zouhair Odeh Amarin

Abstract

Hysterectomy is a major operation and is as old as time. This chapter touches briefly on the history of this procedure, its present aspects and general advice for these women who may need a hysterectomy, and finally the direction of new developments about it.

Keywords: hysterectomy, vaginal hysterectomy, abdominal hysterectomy, laparoscopic hysterectomy, robotic hysterectomy

1. Introduction

Hysterectomy is the surgical removal of the uterus and, in some circumstances, the ovaries, cervix, fallopian tubes and supporting tissues. It ranks, just behind cesarean section, as the second most common surgery among women, and is the most common non-pregnancy-related major surgery performed on women worldwide.

Hysterectomy is a major surgical procedure that has risks and benefits, and may be classified as abdominal and vaginal according to the route of access. The abdominal route may be through conventional laparotomy, laparoscopy or robotic surgery, or vaginal hysterectomy through the superior part of the vagina. Occasionally both routes are used in combination.

2. Indications

The indications for hysterectomy include benign conditions such as dysfunctional uterine bleeding, uterine fibroids, endometriosis, adenomyosis and genital prolapse. In addition, it is indicated in cases of gynecological malignancies Of the uterus, ovaries and cervix, and for future malignancy risk-reducing indications, such as cases of BRCA 1 or 2 mutations or Lynch syndrome [1, 2].

3. History

The origin of hysterectomy is obscure, but the first operation was vaginal hysterectomy that reputedly was performed by Soranus of Ephesus in the Greek city of Ephesus around 160 AD for the extirpation of an inverted uterus that had become gangrenous [3].

Historically, time passed with no clear record of advancement until the beginning of the 19th century. Lauvariol of France is credited for performing the first vaginal hysterectomy, followed by Baudelocque, who artificially prolapsed and then cut away the uterus and its appendages [3].

It was at the beginning of the 19th century too, in 1809, that the world's first abdominal surgery was performed on a kitchen table. The operator was Ephraim McDowell from Danville, Kentucky. He removed an ovarian cyst that weighed 10.2 k. The patient survived [3].

Early procedures were performed without anesthesia, with some milk, brandy and prayers for some comfort, but the performance of medical procedures that caused intolerable pain to patients was technically unfeasible until anesthesia became part of the surgery. It enabled patients to undergo an operation safely without experiencing severe distress and intolerable pain.

By 1831, ether, nitrous oxide and chloroform had been discovered, albeit not applied medically yet. The first use of anesthesia in surgery was by Crawford Long of Georgia who, in 1842, used nitrous oxide on a very limited number of minor surgical cases. A few years later anesthesia was considered and implemented as a major breakthrough [3].

Of interest is the fact that dentistry was the first profession to use anesthesia, A Connecticut dentist, Horace Wells, in 1844, tested nitrous oxide by having his own tooth removed whilst under the influence of the gas. Wells' dental student, William Morton introduced ether to dental procedures in 1846, and is regarded as the world's first anesthetist, after the name 'anesthesia' was suggested by Oliver Holmes [3].

James Simpson of Edinburgh employed anesthesia in childbirth. This was condemned by the Calvinist Church as being against its beliefs. Because of its odor and long induction period, Simpson abandoned ether in favor of chloroform, which was favored in Europe until its hepatic toxicity became clear. Of interest is the fact that John Snow used it for Queen Victoria's delivery of Princess Charlotte with no apparent ill effects [4].

With the new developments in medicine, in general, anesthesia and surgery in particular, continued their advancements and refinements. The lower transverse abdominal incision along the pubic hairline was introduced by Johannes Pfannenstiel of Breslau in the 1920s. Harry Reich performed the first laparoscopic hysterectomy in Kingston, Pennsylvania in 1988 [5, 6].

4. Types

There are different types of hysterectomy. A subtotal hysterectomy, also known as supracervical hysterectomy, removes the uterus and leaves the cervix intact. A small proportion of patients undergoing subtotal hysterectomy continue to have cyclical bleeding until menopause [7, 8].

To minimize the possibility of this, the procedure of supracervical hysterectomy is combined with a reverse cone excision of the endocervical endometrium to avoid having very light menstruation.

A total hysterectomy removes the uterus and cervix. A radical hysterectomy may be indicated in certain cases of malignancy where the uterus, cervix and part of the vagina, ovaries, fallopian tubes, and nearby lymph nodes are removed.

A peripartum hysterectomy or emergency peripartum hysterectomy is a life-saving procedure to remove the uterus after 20 weeks of gestation, occurring during or after delivery or during the puerperium due to severe hemorrhage that fails to respond to conservative medical therapy and other modalities. Uterine atony and morbid placentation are the leading abnormalities [9–11].

Compared with non-obstetric hysterectomy, peripartum hysterectomy is associated with a six-fold increase in blood loss, and a 25-fold increase in mortality due to the increased incidence of coagulopathies and other perioperative complications [12].

5. Techniques

Regarding hysterectomy techniques, the procedure can be performed through the vagina, the abdomen or by laparoscopy. The decision will depend on the indication for the operation, past abdominal surgery, current medical conditions, weight, available equipment and surgeon's expertise.

Abdominal hysterectomy, also known as traditional open surgery, is performed through an abdominal incision, mostly by Pfannenstiel incision, and less frequently through an up and down incision. It is more recommended in cases of very large uterus, in cases of malignancies, and associations with other organ pathologies. This traditional approach is associated with relatively more post-operative pain and slightly longer hospital stay.

At vaginal hysterectomy the uterus is excised through an incision at the vaginal vault, thus avoiding an abdominal incision. This procedure is preferred in cases of uterine prolapse, vaginal walls laxity, stress incontinence and deficient perineum. To be eligible for a vaginal hysterectomy, the uterus must be of a certain size as it is not very suitable in cases of large pelvic masses and suspected malignancies.

Laparoscopic hysterectomy is a minimally invasive procedure using laparoscopic surgery where the uterus is removed through the vagina. The procedure seems to combine "the best of both worlds". It is associated with fewer complications in the suitably selected cases and the availability of adequate instruments, surgical expertise and assistance.

Robotic hysterectomy is laparoscopic surgery that is aided by a robot that allows the performance of more complex procedures with better precision. The technology includes specialized arms for instrument holding, a camera, and a magnified screen and a console. This allows a greater range of motion and dexterity for better access to the area of interest. Recovery is similar to traditional laparoscopic surgery.

6. Implications and general advice

The hospital stay after hysterectomy is usually 3 days. Postoperatively, prophylactic anticoagulation should be administered for about 10 days, and may be for longer in cases of hysterectomy due to cancer. Post hysterectomy, it may take 4–6 weeks to recover. The age and overall health will influence recovery time. In general, after a hysterectomy, an individual should not drive for 2 weeks, and not lift heavy objects for 6 weeks. Recovery may be aided by gentle exercise and gentle cleaning of the abdominal surgical incision. At follow-up, except for subtotal hysterectomy, the vaginal vault is checked for any granulation tissue, and if present it could be touched with silver nitrate.

When deciding on the route of hysterectomy, it has to be taken into account that, compared with abdominal hysterectomy, vaginal hysterectomy, as well as laparoscopic hysterectomy, are associated with less blood loss, shorter hospital stay, less post-operative pain, quicker return to usual activities and fess abdominal incisional infections [13–15].

Because of these findings, a recent review advocated that vaginal hysterectomy is preferable to abdominal hysterectomy. Furthermore, when vaginal hysterectomy is neither advisable nor practical, then laparoscopic hysterectomy should be considered [6].

In general, vaginal hysterectomy is not as expensive as abdominal hysterectomy, but it can be more difficult if adnexal masses are present, or in women with previous abdominal surgery or endometriosis. In addition, vaginal hysterectomy can be more challenging in cases of minimal uterine descent and patients with a narrow sub-pubic arch.

The adoption of the laparoscopic approach for the performance of hysterectomy has been slow. This, in part, has been attributed to the need for specialized highly technical equipment that is more delicate than those used in conventional surgery, and is in more need for routine maintenance. In addition, training programs lack a requirement that trainees need to have performed a certain number of laparoscopic procedures before graduating [16, 17].

For postoperative care, the best analgesic regimens are those that offer broad coverage, safe and are easy to administer. For moderate to severe pain, a centrally acting synthetic opioid analgesic with lower opiate-like dependence than Morphine would be appropriate. Non-steroidal anti-inflammatory drugs that possess analgesic and anti-pyretic activity are equally suitable. For nausea and vomiting patients are given the appropriate prophylactic and therapeutic antiemetics, such as dexamethasone and ondansetron [18–20].

After laparoscopic hysterectomy, it is normal to have some shoulder or back pain that is caused by the pneumoperitoneum. Patients tend to get tired easily or have less energy that lasts for several weeks after surgery, and may take about 4 to 6 weeks to fully recover. It's important to avoid lifting while recovering. Patients are advised to be active where walking is a good choice, and to rest when feeling tired. Diet should be normal. In cases of an upset stomach, bland, low-fat foods and yogurt is advisable. Drinking plenty of water may avoid constipation.

To avoid venous thromboembolism, antiplatelet medication, in the form of acetylsalicylic acid, or low molecular heparin should be prescribed.

Abdominal incisions could be washed daily with warm, soapy water, and patted dry. Hydrogen peroxide or alcohol should be avoided as they can slow wound healing. The area may be covered with a gauze bandage that should be changed daily, if it oozes any discharge or rubs against clothing.

Follow-up after hysterectomy is mandatory. Light vaginal bleeding is not unusual. Patients should use sanitary pads if needed and avoid vaginal douches or the use of tampons. Intercourse is not allowed for six weeks, and after being cleared at the follow-up check.

Bilateral oophorectomy in premenopausal women would cause an abrupt loss of ovarian hormones which may alter some fundamental aging processes at the cellular and system levels [21]. An association of bilateral oophorectomy with increased DNA methylation has been reported [22].

Other than DNA methylation studies, further new research is needed to investigate the association of bilateral oophorectomy with aging using brain imaging, in addition to physical and functional measures of balance, gait, limb strength, cognitive function, markers of Alzheimer's disease and of cerebrovascular disease [23].

7. Present day issues

Nowadays, newer surgical options and techniques include laparoscopic incisions, single umbilical incisions, and robotic-assisted procedures. Such minimally-invasive hysterectomy approaches require a shorter hospital stay, with full recovery in four to six weeks.

Regarding hysterectomy for heavy and prolonged menstruation, endometrial curettage has been proven ineffective as a treatment as a reduction in bleeding may last for only one menstrual period and not after this. Curettage is utilized as a diagnostic procedure to determine the cause of the heavy bleeding.

The need to curette the uterus for histopathological purposes could be replaced by endometrial sampling where a fine plastic tube is passed inside the uterine cavity as an outpatient procedure. Vaginal ultrasound and hysteroscopy are the most commonly used procedures for reaching a histopathological diagnosis.

Endometrial ablation of the uterus is a day procedure, where a slightly lower proportion of women perceive improvement in bleeding symptoms, but it results in an improvement in pictorial blood loss assessment charts compared to their baseline score. Repeat surgery resulting from the failure of the initial treatment is more likely to be required after endometrial ablation than after hysterectomy, and the satisfaction rate is lower after endometrial ablation [24].

Regarding morbidity, it is more likely after hysterectomy. Women after endometrial ablation are less likely to experience sepsis, blood transfusion, pyrexia, vault hematoma and wound hematoma before hospital discharge, and a higher rate of infection after hospital discharge [24].

Unfortunately, not many clinicians are proficient in performing endometrial ablation, Alternatives to surgery include tranexamic acid in the first few days of heavy bleeding each month, progestogen tablets and progesterone impregnated intrauterine devices. In additions oral contraceptive pills and anti-prostaglandins may result in a sizable reduction in bleeding.

Second to menorrhagia, the most common reason for the hysterectomy is the presence of fibroids. Alternatives to hysterectomy that should be considered are laparoscopic myomectomy, myolysis and laparoscopic uterine artery ligation, and radiological uterine artery embolization. Hysterectomy remains an option for a small percentage where other modalities would have failed.

8. Future considerations

Worldwide, there are so many hysterectomized women, where developed countries have higher hysterectomy rates than their developing counterparts. There are some alternatives to hysterectomy for patients with heavy bleeding and for fibroids to decrease the frequency of non-hysterectomy solutions for these patients. There is a need for better training programs for all gynecologists about the alternative methods and new techniques that require more skill. Although, hysterectomy has full success in dealing with abnormal and heavy uterine bleeding and fibroids, it is associated with certain morbidity and, to a much lesser degree, mortality.

Finally, the vast majority of patients do not want to have a hysterectomy. All important information should be given to them about alternative procedures. Patients can decide themselves what is best for them.

Author details

Zouhair Odeh Amarin
Department of Obstetrics and Gynecology, Jordan University of Science and Technology, Jordan

*Address all correspondence to: zoamarin@hotmail.com

References

[1] Jones HW III. Abdominal hysterectomy. In: Rock J, Jones H III, editors. TeLinde's Operative Gynecology. 10th ed. Wolters Kluwer Health: Lippincott Williams & Wilkins; 2008. pp. 727-744

[2] Kovac RS. Vaginal hysterectomy. In: Rock J, Jones H III, editors. TeLinde's Operative Gynecology. 10th ed. Wolters Kluwer Health: Lippincott Williams & Wilkins; 2008. pp. 744-763

[3] Sutton C. Hysterectomy: A historical perspective. Baillière's Clinical Obstetrics and Gynaecology. 1997;**11**(1):1-22 The world's first hysterectomy was performed by Clay in his consulting rooms in Piccadilly, Manchester, England in 1843. The patient did not survive. In: 1853 Ellis Burnham from Lowell, Massachusetts performed the first successful abdominal hysterectomy with a patient surviving (4)

[4] Benrubi GI. History of hysterectomy. Journal of the Florida Medical Association. 1988;**75**(8):533-538

[5] Harris WJ, Daniell JF. Early complications of laparoscopic hysterectomy. Obstetrical & Gynecological Survey. 1996;**51**:559-567

[6] Härkki-Siren P, Sjöberg J, Kurki T. Major complications of laparoscopy: A follow-up Finnish study. Obstetrics and Gynecology. 1999;**94**:94-98

[7] Van der Stege JG, van Beek JJ. Problems related to the cervical stump at follow-up in laparoscopic supracervical hysterectomy. JSLS: Journal of the Society of Laparoendoscopic Surgeons. 1999;**3**:5-7

[8] Nisolle M, Donnez J. Subtotal hysterectomy in patients with endometriosis-an option. Fertility and Sterility. 1997;**67**:1185-1187

[9] Whiteman MK, Kalian E, Hillis SD, et al. Incidence and determinants of peripartum hysterectomy. Obstetrics and Gynecology. 2006;**108**:1486-1492

[10] Knight M, on behalf of UKOSS. Peripartum hysterectomy in the UK: Management and outcomes of the associated haemorrhage. BJOG: An International Journal of Obstetrics and Gynaecology. 2007;**114**:1380-1387

[11] Awan N, Bennett MJ, Walters WAW. Emergency peripartum hysterectomy: A 10-year review at the Royal Hospital for women, Sydney. The Australian and New Zealand Journal of Obstetrics and Gynaecology. 2011;**51**:210-215

[12] Wright JD, Devine P, Shah M, et al. Morbidity and mortality of peripartum hysterectomy. Obstetrics and Gynecology. Jun 2010;**115**(6):1187-1193

[13] Clayton RD. Hysterectomy. Best Practice & Research. Clinical Obstetrics & Gynaecology. 2006;**20**:73-87

[14] Johnson N, Barlow D, Lethaby A, et al. Surgical approach to hysterectomy for benign gynaecological disease. Cochrane Database of Systematic Reviews. 2006;**2**:CD003677

[15] Johnson N, Barlow D, Lethaby A, et al. Methods of hysterectomy: Systematic review and meta-analysis of randomised controlled trials. BMJ. 2005;**330**:1478

[16] Reich H. Total laparoscopic hysterectomy: Indications, techniques and outcomes. Current Opinion in Obstetrics & Gynecology. 2007;**19**:337-344

[17] Englund M, Robson S. Why has the acceptance of laparoscopic hysterectomy been slow? Results of an anonymous survey of Australian gynecologists. Journal of Minimally Invasive Gynecology. 2007;**14**:724-728

[18] Einarsson J, Suzuki Y. Total laparoscopic hysterectomy: 10 steps toward a successful procedure. Rev. Obstetrics and Gynecology. 2009;**2**(1):57-64

[19] Gan TJ. Risk factors for postoperative nausea and vomiting. Anesthesia and Analgesia. 2006;**102**:1884-1898

[20] Einarsson JI, Audbergsson BO, Thorsteinsson A. Scopolamine for prevention of postoperative nausea in gynecologic laparoscopy, a randomized trial. Journal of Minimally Invasive Gynecology. 2008;**15**:26-31

[21] Rocca WA, Gazzuola-Rocca L, Smith CY, Grossardt BR, Faubion SS, Shuster LT, et al. Accelerated accumulation of multimorbidity after bilateral oophorectomy: A population-based cohort study. Mayo Clinic Proceedings. 2016;**91**:1577-1589. DOI: 10.1016/j.mayocp.2016.08.002

[22] Levine ME, Lu AT, Chen BH, Hernandez DG, Singleton AB, Ferrucci L, et al. Menopause accelerates biological aging. Proceedings of the National Academy of Sciences. 2016;**113**:9327-9332

[23] Rocca WA, Gazzuola Rocca L, Smith CY, Grossardt BR, Faubion SS, Shuster LT, et al. Loss of ovarian hormones and accelerated somatic and mental aging. Physiology (Bethesda, Md.). 2018;**33**(6):374-383. DOI: 10.1152/physiol.00024.2018

[24] Fergusson RJ, Bofill Rodriguez M, Lethaby A, Farquhar C. Endometrial resection and ablation versus hysterectomy for heavy menstrual bleeding. Cochrane Database of Systematic Reviews. 2019;**8**(8):CD000329. DOI: 10.1002/14651858.CD000329.pub3 Update in: Cochrane Database Syst Rev. 2021 Feb 23

Chapter 2

From Open to Minimally Invasive: The Sacrocolpopexy

Adriana Fulginiti, Frank Borao, Martin Michalewski and Robert A. Graebe

Abstract

With an increased demand for pelvic organ prolapse surgeries as the population ages, mesh-related osteomyelitis will become more prevalent. This case series enriches the paucity of data on management options for delayed osteomyelitis related to pelvic organ prolapse mesh. A literature review revealed no case reports of delayed onset osteomyelitis presenting up to a decade after colpopexy mesh placement. We present three cases of delayed osteomyelitis, their presentation, diagnosis and management at a tertiary academic referral center. Patients presented between 1 and 10 years after mesh colpopexy. Three different mesh materials were utilized during the initial procedures: Restorelle Y, Gynamesh and Gore-Tex mesh. The first case demonstrates failed expectant management with eventual surgical intervention on a medically compromised patient. The two subsequent cases describe elective complete mesh resection after several prior failed mesh revision attempts. This short case series and literature review illustrates that mesh-related osteomyelitis after a remote sacrocolpopexy carries significant morbidity. Mesh removal by means of minimally invasive surgery in the hands of an experienced surgical team utilizing DaVinci Robotic System is a good option and may lead to best patient outcomes.

Keywords: Sacrocolpopexy, mesh, Urogynecology, robotic, osteomyelitis, erosion

1. Introduction

Arthure first described a method of fixating the prolapsed uterus to the sacral promontory in 1957 [1] and Lane introduced the concept of vaginal apex or uterine suspension to the sacral promontory using an intervening graft in 1962 [2]. The abdominal sacrocolpopexy (ASC) is the most durable repair for advanced pelvic organ prolapse (POP) and became the gold standard surgical treatment for apical vaginal defects, with long-term success rates of 78–100% [3–6]. Although ASC was established as the most durable operation, the morbidity associated with laparotomy limited its broad use especially in the elderly, obese or in women with significant medical comorbidities [5, 7]. In the last two decades, minimally invasive approaches have been widely accepted as an alternative option to ASC [8–10]. Laparoscopic sacrocolpopexy (LSC) was first reported in 1994 by Nezhat [11]. Robotic Assisted Sacrocolpopexy (RAS) was described a decade later by DiMarco [12] in 2004. Since the Food and Drug Administration (FDA) approval of the DaVinci Surgical system (Intuitive Surgical, Inc., Sunnyvale, CA) for gynecological operations in 2005, it has become a fundamental part of the armamentarium in complex pelvic floor procedures [13].

Compared to the abdominal route, minimally invasive sacrocolpopexies are more costly and can be more time consuming in the inexperienced hands. Level I evidence from as early as 2012 supported LSC as the lower-risk option with improved anatomic and subjective outcomes, lower recurrence rates, less post-operative dyspareunia, less blood loss and faster recovery [4, 7, 14, 15]. Maher et al.'s randomized clinical trial demonstrated shorter hospital stay, earlier return to daily activity, improved anatomical outcomes, and less graft-related complications. There were also less re-interventions and related hospital costs, which ultimately outweighed longer operation times [15].

The limitation to wide acceptance of laparoscopic reconstructive pelvic surgery was the need for advanced surgical skill to dissect the pre-sacral space and suture mesh graft to the vagina and sacrum, which many surgeons found too arduous or time consuming to perform. Data shows that approximately 30 LSCs need to be performed to achieve an operation time comparable to an experienced surgeon, and about 60 are needed to obtain similar complication rates [7]. Long-term evidence across all surgical disciplines unequivocally shows that outcomes of high volume surgeons are superior, with lower complication rates [16, 17].

The number of women undergoing Pelvic Organ Prolapse (POP) procedures is estimated at 400,000 annually in the U.S. and an additional 260,000 for stress urinary incontinence (SUI) [18–20]. Over 50% of women over 65 years have some form of urinary incontinence. It is predicted that by 2030, about 20% of the U.S. population will be within this age group, increased from 13% in 2010 [21]. With aging demographics, the national burden related to pelvic floor disorders (PFD), decreased quality of life, and demand for pelvic floor surgeries is expected to increase. In 2010 there were 1,218,371 new pelvic floor-related patient visits in the U.S. [22]. The U.S. Census and NHANES data estimates that the number of women with PFD is expected to reach 43.8 million by 2050 [23]. With more cases of intra-abdominally placed mesh for POP, and with robotic advancements, it is expected that there will be an increased number of complications such as lumbosacral osteomyelitis [20]. Mesh associated osteomyelitis has been reported in only a few cases, with none presenting up to a decade after mesh placement.

Prosthetic vaginal mesh for POP repairs was introduced in the 1990s, and became liberally used in the mid 2000s, aiming to replace long and complex intra-abdominal procedures. In 2004 FDA approved vaginal meshes as POP repair kits. This resulted in standardization of surgical techniques across the U.S. and allowed for more robust research [24, 25]. Introduced by American Medical Systems (San Jose, CA), Apogee and Perigee systems were the first ready-to-use pelvic mesh repair kits commercially available in 2005 [24]. Shortly after they were followed by the most widely used Gynacare Ethicon's Prolift kits (Johnson and Johnson, Sommerville NJ) and many others such as C.R. Bard, Boston Scientific, Coloplast, and Cook Medical [24, 25]. Mesh kits were brought to the market relatively fast, and as the Gartner curve shows with most innovations, industry hype and corporate avarice lead to mass marketing, and drawbacks become clear when use of mesh became more widespread [26]. Between 2005 and 2010 in the U.S., J&J Ethicon's Gynacare division sold over $1 Billion worth of female POP repair mesh products alone.

Direct and aggressive marketing by large corporation sales-representatives to inadequately trained in pelvic reconstructive surgery ObGyns and general Urologists led to inappropriate procedures. Often after a minimal "training course" and/or cadaver lab, many physicians became "mesh repair specialists" advertised by the product manufacturer. Regretfully, repairs for prophylactic reasons or due to peer pressure, and use of mesh simply to boost revenue from anterior-posterior repairs became common. Increased complication rates and reports of significant patient morbidity became evident. Bleeding (0–3%), visceral injury (1–4%), urinary infection (0–19%), graft erosion (0–30%), and fistula formation (1%) led to FDA review of Urogynecologic mesh products [19, 27]. There was a five-fold increased complication rate from 2005 to 2007 compared to the previous three years [19]. From October 2008 to 2011, surgical mesh outcomes were scrutinized, revealing an additional 2874 reports of adverse events with POP mesh repairs, and 1371 with stress urinary incontinence (SUI) repairs, resulting in the FDA advisory warning: "complications of POP repairs with mesh are not rare and may be difficult to treat" [19].

The most frequently reported issues were urinary tract infections (UTI), urinary retention, mesh erosion, dyspareunia, bleeding, and organ perforation. More than half of women with erosion from non-absorbable synthetic mesh required surgical removal [19, 28–30]. There were seven reported deaths from POP repairs [19]. The FDA conducted a scientific literature review from 1996 to 2011, which showed that symptomatic results or quality of life were not improved with use of mesh versus the traditional native repair [31]. In light of this, the FDA reclassified mesh for transvaginal repair from Class II to Class III "High Risk", which required manufacturers to submit premarket approval applications [19]. In 2012, J&J Ethicon and C.R. Bard were first to voluntarily remove their POP mesh kits from the markets due to increased litigation and diminishing profits [18, 32]. Ethicon's Gynemesh and Coloplast's Restorelle are still in use, although with a future still uncertain [19].

Women are exposed to lawsuit advertisements in various media focused on complications of surgical mesh, and presented with tragic, yet often, anecdotal stories [26, 33, 34]. While acknowledging these warnings, many organizations have missed the opportunity to proactively confront the vaginal mesh debate. Instead of gathering surgeons and industry together to improve the use of mesh, initiate protocols for selecting optimal surgical candidates, and standardize recommendations for surgeon credentialing, pelvic mesh kit manufacturers have succumbed to the bans and quickly settled ensuing tort case law suits. The biggest companies such as Johnson & Johnson moved towards more lucrative "new" non-surgical treatment options such as anti-incontinence vaginal inserts and pessaries. Treatments became focused on pelvic floor muscle strengthening with adjunctive therapies, vaginal cones, kegel chairs, laser vaginal rejuvenation and electrical muscle stimulation devices whose benefits are often difficult to substantiate [35, 36]. From vaginal pessaries first described in 1550 BC [20], the market has expanded to include vaginal rings, self-powered wireless urinary incontinence sensors for disposable diapers [37], and intra-vaginal inserts. Adult diapers has become the next multi-billion dollar industry as they were aggressively advertised and fast out-paced infant diaper sales in the U.S. [35]. In 2012, the North American market for adult incontinence pads and diapers sold 11 billion units worth $4.42 billion [38]. Major personal care brands such as Depend, Poise, and Tena are aimed to remove the social stigmatism around incontinence, with advertisement campaigns and product launches targeting the boomer generation [38]. Young athletes and celebrities are used in late-night advertisements to influence women of all ages [31, 33, 34, 38].

The first decade of the twenty-first century was also a time of fast-paced technological advancement. With increased equipment availability and acceptance within the surgical community of DaVinci robotic surgical systems in mid 2000s, the use of robotic technology made LSC a more accessible procedure. These advancements permitted precise and intuitive movements, allowing suturing of mesh to the vagina with relative ease for more practitioners [3, 7, 39, 40]. Improved ergonomics and the three-dimensional viewing of the robotic system provided better visualization of tissue planes and vasculature near the sacral promontory, allowing for faster dissection and overall safer procedures with less blood loss and better outcomes [3]. Robotic wristed instruments improved dexterity, requiring fewer cases to gain surgical competence, and became more attractive in a wider number of surgical theaters [7, 39, 40]. There is paucity of data comparing patient outcomes between laparoscopic and robotic assisted sacrocolpopexies (RAS). The randomized controlled ACCESS trial demonstrated that RAS are more costly than LSCs ($19,616 vs. $11,573, $p < 0.001$) [3, 7] with no difference in procedure time (225 vs. 246 min $p = 0.110$), anatomical outcomes, pelvic floor function, or quality of life [3, 7].

While vaginal mesh complications are extensively researched and publicized, research data of intra-abdominally placed mesh for pelvic floor repairs issues are obscure [8, 40, 41]. Descriptions of mesh problems associated with placement by endoscopic procedures are even more rare. Available data pertains to the risks that are mostly those specific to laparoscopy, use of general anesthesia, pneumoperitoneum and prolonged Trendelenburg positioning [42, 43]. Complications of vaginal POP repairs with mesh are widely reported, however, what is attributable to poor technique versus mesh itself is debatable. Published data from self-proclaimed "mesh removal experts" confirm this. Margulies et al. (a vocal critic of vaginal mesh and a prominent plaintiff expert), identified mesh folding at the time of mesh excision surgery in 69% of patients who had their mesh removed due to dyspareunia [44]. During Crosby's surgeries for mesh removal, he also found that mesh to be folded or had significant tension in 70% of his patients [45].

Cho et al. performed a large case review to compare LSC to the traditional open procedure. There were no significant intraoperative complications other than a 1.08% risk of blood transfusion, and a low rate of postoperative complications (8% constipation, 4% lower abdominal discomfort, 5% urge incontinence, 4% vaginal spotting, and less than 3% for all other complications) [43]. Meticulous mesh placement and improved visualization resulted in good long-term outcomes (0% relapse rate at 1 year) [20]. 98.8% of women were satisfied with their surgical outcome, with no reports of sexual dysfunction [43]. Altogether, these results show that the minimally invasive approach has better outcomes comparable to the abdominal approach, and is also significantly safer and more efficient [46]. In view of medico-legal climate and with politically prevailing negative opinions of vaginal mesh, abdominally placed mesh via minimally invasive surgery for POP is safe, durable, and currently the best option. As in any mesh/implant surgery, patient selection, surgical field sterility, avoidance of excessive electrocautery, clear planes of dissection, meticulous hemostasis and proper mesh placement are of the uttermost importance [44, 45].

With the vaginal mesh industry on hold, many prominent pelvic surgeons reverted to intra-abdominal repairs. The options range from the classic sacrocolpopexy in which the vaginal cuff after hysterectomy is affixed to the anterior longitudinal ligament (ALL) with permanent sutures and Y-shaped mesh graft [9, 47], to uteropexy to preserve fertility [47]. These repairs can be done with sutures, with or without mesh graft [9, 47]. Variants of the repair include sacral cervicocolpopexy, now the most commonly utilized by FPMRS specialists in the U.S., in which preservation of the cervical stump during hysterectomy facilitates suturing of the vaginal apex to ligaments [10]. This procedure is easier and safer, reduces operating times, and decreases the risk of mesh complications five fold [10]. Other options are sacrocolpoperineopexy [10] or modification of anterior or posterior rectopexy [48]. The choice of the procedure depends on patient site-specific defects and the comfort of the operating surgeon. There is also colpopectopexy, a modification of the apical vaginal suspension where the lateral aspects of the illiopectineal ligaments are used for unilateral or bilateral fixation of prolapsing vagina, which gained some hold first in Europe and later in the.

U.S. [49] (Case 2). Advancements in MIS, robotics and laparoscopy continue with the fast pacing introduction of better visualization systems, artificial intelligence, machine learning, computer enhanced surgery and integration of imaging studies into the live surgical field.

Complications of Minimally Invasive Surgery (MIS) with mesh for POP, diagnostic modalities, findings and management protocols are under-publicized. In 2011, Smith and Davila proposed a vaginal approach on how to manage small versus large mesh exposures, mesh contractions and infection, and also recommended preventative strategies [50]. However, reports are still lacking on how to manage infected mesh deep in the sacral region. Our three cases demonstrate that laparoscopic and robotic approaches to intra-abdominal mesh complications are feasible and can be utilized in a safe, efficient, and effective manner in the proper surgical setting. The described cases attempt to shed light on delayed onset osteomyelitis of the lumbosacral vertebrae, one of the rarely reported, but morbid complications of sacrocolpopexy. Its presentation, complications, and complexity of the intraoperative field are reviewed. As the use of permanent sutures and mesh implants in the vicinity of ligaments and bone increases, potential for osteomyelitis will increase. FPMRS surgeons applying mesh to the intra-peritoneal cavity must be extra vigilant in timely recognition and treatment of this once rare condition [14, 27].

A literature search showed that there is no case report of delayed onset osteomyelitis presenting up to a decade after mesh placement. We present three cases of osteomyelitis including presentation, diagnosis and management from a tertiary academic referral center. Patients presented between 1 and 10 years after mesh colpopexy procedure. Three different mesh materials were utilized during the initial POP repair procedures: Restorelle Y, Gynamesh and Gore-tex mesh.

The first case demonstrates failed expectant management followed by surgical intervention on a medically compromised patient, whereas the two subsequent cases describe elective surgical repairs undertaken after several prior failed mesh removal attempts. All cases were successfully managed by a multidisciplinary surgical team, completely resecting infected meshs utilizing DaVinci Xi Robotic System.

Case 1: Chronic urinary tract infection and back pain, vaginal malodorous discharge and pulmonary embolism.

74yo white female with a history of 4th degree uterovaginal prolapse who underwent DaVinci assisted laparoscopic sacral colpopexy and laparoscopic supracervical hysterectomy (LSC/LSH/BSO) with Restorelle Y polypropylene mesh (Coloplast) in 2015. Eighteen months after surgery the patient presented to a local emergency room with lower back and abdominal pain. She was diagnosed with UTI and discharged home on oral antibiotics. She presented 1 month later to our institution with fever and a history of chronic UTI, worsening back pain and generalized weakness. She was admitted by for intravenous antibiotics with presumptive diagnosis of pyelonephritis complicated by urosepsis. During her workup it was discovered that she also had a pulmonary embolism and was treated accordingly.

Computed Tomography (CT) scan showed hyper-enhancement of the lumbar sacral joints L5 to S1, with Magnetic Resonance Imaging (MRI) noted a well-defined enhancing fistulous tract from the lumbosacral region to the vaginal space consistent with discitis and osteomyelitis (**Figure 1A** and **B**). The patient's mental status was slightly impaired either due to age, delirium from nicotine withdrawal, or current medical condition. She was a heavy lifetime smoker with history of chronic obstructive pulmonary disease (COPD), a non-compliant patient and poor historian. Her pulmonary embolus was treated, she was kept on IV antibiotics for the discitis, the fever subsided, and the patient condition was stabilized. She then developed a new onset of malodorous vaginal discharge. Patient's family reported a

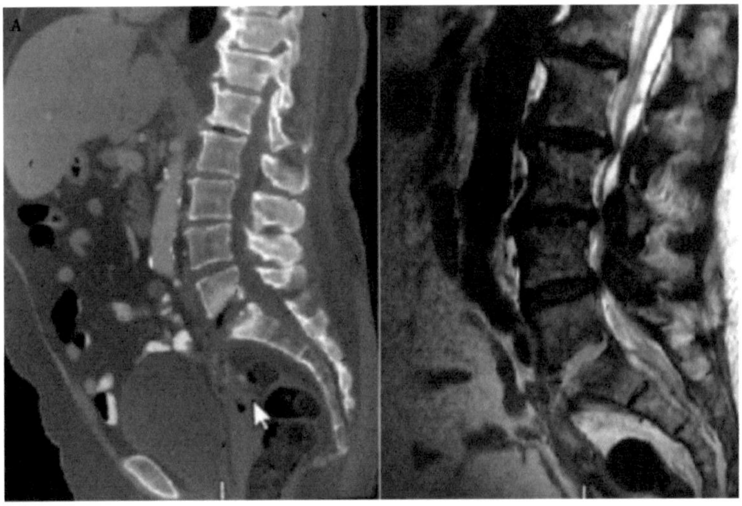

Figure 1.
(A and B) MRI showing discitis and osteomyelitis.

history of prior POP mesh repair. Urogynecologic and Spine surgeons were consulted at that time and vaginal examination showed apical abscess with copious foul discharge.

Diagnosis of a lumbosacral-peritoneal-vaginal fistula tract with mesh erosion was made. Despite 2 weeks of intravenous (IV) broad-spectrum antibiotic therapy, there was lack of improvement in pain, copious daily drainage increased and lumbosacral osteomyelitis worsened. Patient had developed local neurological deficits in the lower extremities compromising her ability to stand up and she could no longer walk. Spine surgical intervention became urgent and despite serious medical comorbidities, in consultation with General surgery and Urogynecology, it was determined that surgical removal of the infected mesh, fistula resection, abscess evacuation, and bone debridement could no longer be further delayed.

Intra-operatively, a vaginal fistulous connection was identified when a probe was passed through the vagina and was visible intra-abdominally to the pre-sacral lumbar bone space (**Figure 2A**). Using DaVinci assisted laparoscopy, adhesions were freed of the involved bowel, and the infected mesh was removed and abscess drained (**Figure 2B**). The bladder and ureter were dissected with illuminated stents in place. Bone debridement was performed and osteopromotive materials were grafted onto the L4 to S1 posterior lumbar region by Spine and Vascular Surgeon, who dissected and patch repaired the left common iliac vein in the process to completely remove mesh from the lumbosacral area. Total operating time of 180 min. The patient was kept on IV antibiotics and anticoagulation for 6 weeks postoperatively while recovering at a nursing facility. She was home in 6 weeks time living independently. Unfortunately she was a heavy smoker with poor hygiene and severe COPD that succumbed to pulmonary complications about 9 months later, albeit unrelated to her surgery.

Case 2: Pelvic pain with persistant right groin/inguinal skin draining sinus tract. History of four failed fistula repairs, ventral and inguinal hernia.

A 70 year-old white female presenting with a right groin/inguinal draining sinus tract and ventral hernia complaining of pelvic and abdominal pain. She had a history of a total abdominal hysterectomy and an open colpopectopexy with Gore-Tex mesh performed in 2005. Subsequently, over the past 5 years she underwent multiple partial mesh revisions and three failed open peritoneo-cutaneous fistula tract

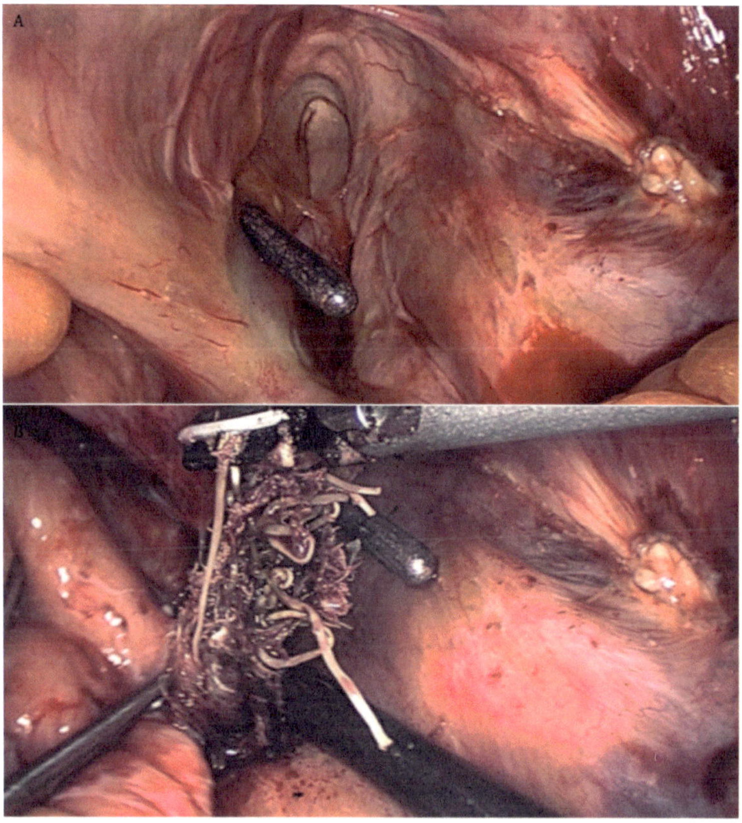

Figure 2.
(A) Probe in fistula canal tracking to ischiopubic bone and iliopectineal ligament (laparoscopic view) and (B) mesh removed from vaginal cuff.

repairs. After numerous second opinions, the patient was referred to our center. The patient presented in 2019 with complaints of abdominal, pelvic pain and chronic persistent groin discharge requiring several pads per day, compromising her daily activities. In the few months prior she also developed a painful lower abdominal bulge. Based on physical examination and CT scan, the patient was diagnosed with an eight-centimeter incarcerated ventral hernia (**Figure 3A**) with a patent fistulous tract from the groin to the upper vagina and intraperitoneal space, draining proximal to the bladder (**Figure 3B**).

Elective robotic repair of the incarcerated ventral hernia and mesh resection with fistula repair was performed. Upon laparoscopic entry, extensive adhesions were noted with loops of small bowel in the hernia sac. A right ureteral lighted stent was inserted illuminating the area of the bladder that was involved in the hernia sac. Under direct laparoscopic and cystoscopic guidance a blunt probe was inserted into the right groin sinus tract opening, mapping the fistula tract to the right pubic bone and right iliopectineal ligament immediately adjunct to bladder and right upper vagina.

The ventral and inguinal hernias were reduced and the fistula tract was dissected noting Gore-Tex mesh and suture material adherent to the inner aspect of the iliopubic bone, its periosteum, bladder and vagina (**Figure 3C**). There was a defect found in the right pubic bone approximately three-centimeter in size with granuloma tissue formation on the mesh that was also involving bone (**Figure 3D**). Bone debridement was performed and cultures showed heavy growth of Serratia Marcescens (SM), pathognomonic to nosocomial infections [51].

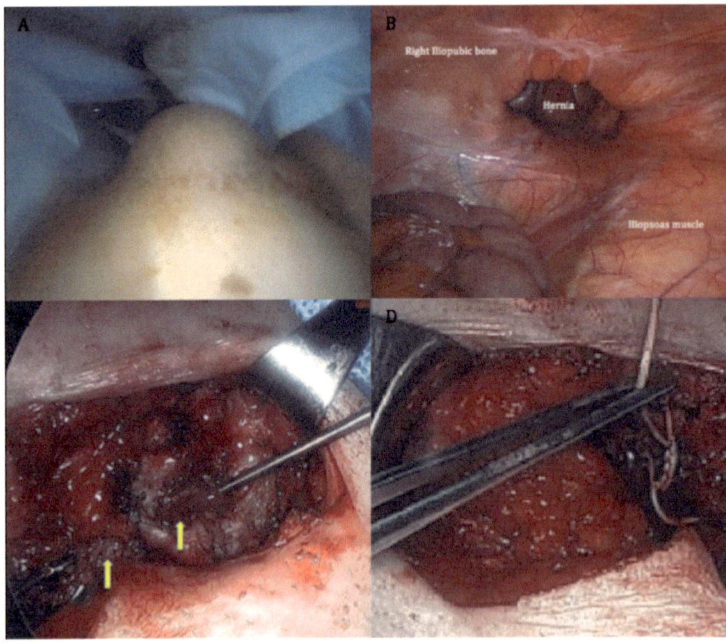

Figure 3.
(A) Outside view of pelvic bulge, (B) laparoscopic view of the hernia after bowel loops reduction, (C) probe in fistula canal tracking to ischiopubic bone and iliopectineal ligament and (D) old Gortex suture material removed from bone defect.

The cutaneoperitoneal tract and vesicovaginal defects were resected and repaired. Cystoscopy with hydrodissection and lighted ureteral stents assured bladder and right ureter integrity. The pubic bone defect was irrigated with antibiotic solution and packed with bone wax. The ventral and right inguinal hernia was repaired creating myofascial advancement flaps. A wound vacuum was applied at a pressure of 125 mmHg (**Figure 4**). Total operating time of 75 min. She was discharged after 24 h.

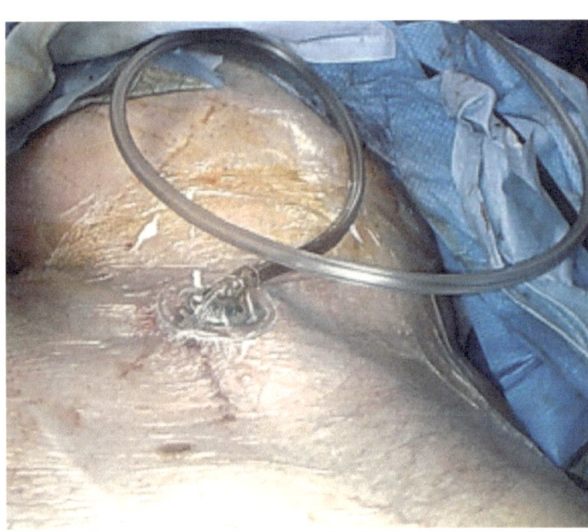

Figure 4.
Wound vacuum at a pressure of 125 mmHg.

Case 3: Pelvic pain, vaginal bleeding, dyspareunia, and chronic vaginal discharge.

52 year-old white female with a history of two prior cesarean sections and DaVinci LSC with Gynecare Y mesh and total laparoscopic hysterectomy (TLH) in 2012 complicated by vaginal apex mesh erosion which caused recurrent vaginal bleeding, dyspareunia and chronic UTI. She had two separate vaginal mesh revisions in 2017 that were further complicated by acute post-surgical intra-abdominal bleeding requiring return to the OR for bladder hematoma evacuation and blood transfusion. The patient presented 2 years later in 2019 complaining of chronic malodorous vaginal discharge, dyspareunia, post-coital bleeding and severe pelvic pain. Vaginal examination revealed copious foul-smelling discharge originating from a necrotic upper vagina with discolored vaginal mesh and pus.

Cultures of the discharge were collected, resulting in heavy growth of Group B Streptococcus and Bacteroides Ovatus. CT scan showed an intra-peritoneal pelvic abscess extending from the presacral space to the upper vagina. Although CT did not identify discitis, an MRI was recommended for evaluation of osteomyelitis that could not be ruled out due to swelling. Since the complications of mesh significantly impacted her quality of life and led to loss of consortium, the patient elected for mesh removal.

Upon laparoscopic evaluation, multiple loops of small bowel were adherent to the pelvic sidewall, occluding the anterior and posterior cul-de-sacs (**Figure 5A**). Frozen pelvis was encountered with dense adhesions of the recto-sigmoid with non-visualization of the sacral promontory. Extensive enterolysis was performed to gain access to the eroded and infected vaginal mesh and pelvic abscess (**Figure 5B**). Multiple loops of the small bowel and rectosigmoid colon were freed from the mesh, presacral space, vagina, bladder and ureter.

Laparoscopic access to the infected Gynecare mesh allowed for evacuation of the intra-abdominal abscess. Once the infected graft was removed, upper vaginectomy and drainage of the pelvic abscess were performed (**Figure 5C**). The anterior longitudinal ligament appeared to be inflamed but not grossly infected. All old fixation sutures were cut and removed.

Early and aggressive intervention in this case prevented progression of upper necrotizing vaginal abscess ascending on the mesh and braided suture (Ethibond)

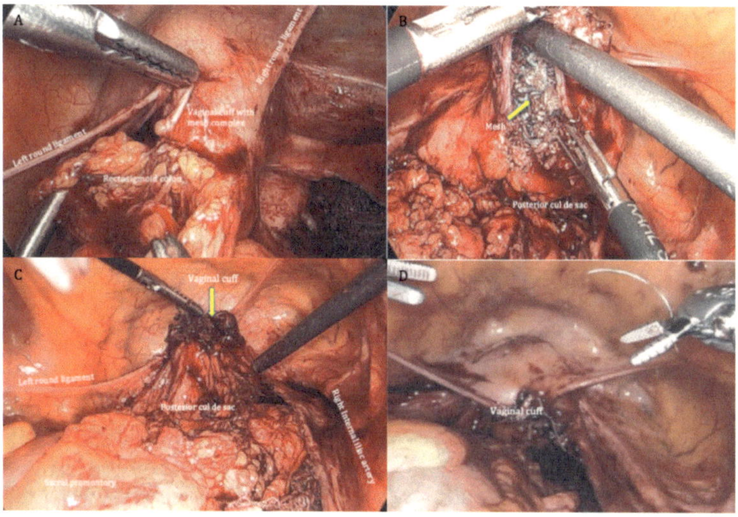

Figure 5.
(A) Dissection of rectosigmoid colon off vaginal cuff/mesh complex, (B) mesh exposed, (C) vaginal cuff with eroded mesh dissected off the pelvic promontory and (D) vaginal cuff closure in layers utilizing the DaVinci Robot.

"ladder" into the anterior longitudinal ligament and periostium of the sacral and lumbar vertebra. DaVinci Xi Robotic system was utilized for the resection of peritoneo-vaginal fistulous tract, entire mesh, upper vaginectomy, and cuff closure (**Figure 5D**).

Integrity of the bladder and rectum were confirmed by cystoscopy and procto-sigmoidoscopy. The patient was discharged home 6 hours later and remains asymptomatic for over 1 year.

2. Discussion

Laparoscopic sacrocolpopexy with synthetic mesh is an effective treatment option for POP with success rates ranging from 78 to 100% [49, 52]. Manufacturer data shows that synthetic mesh can induce an inflammatory process that can result in fibrosis and scarring, distorting normal anatomy and changing the mesh characteristics [45]. Mesh exposure after POP or SUI procedures ranges from 2 to 30% [52], with reoperation rate of 7.9% for apical and 12.7% for other compartments repair as per Cochrane review [51]. Infected and/or exposed mesh can erode into nearby bone and periostium and cause osteomyelitis. Jenson's report states that lumbosacral osteomyelitis and discitis usually occur by hematogenous spread but can also occur from direct inoculation after SCP when bone anchors or permanent sutures are inadvertently placed too deep into the L5-S1 disc space. Mesh exposure is also associated with chronic cigarette smoking, which may have had significance for the patient of Case 1 [53]. Osteomyelitis has been reported to have a median time of presentation of 4 months following a POP procedure [8, 32]. Our cases show that it can present up to 10 years later.

In 1997, Amid et al. classified mesh into different types. Type I mesh are monofilament, flexible and light-weight. They are recommended for most pelvic organ reconstructive procedures because their large pore size greater than 75 mcg allows for tissue integration and for immune cells to scavenge bacteria [54, 55]. Examples are polypropylene Restorelle mesh (used in Case 1), Gynemesh (used in Case 3), Atrium, and Marlex. Type II are microporous with pores less than 10 mcg, such as Gore-Tex (used in Case 2). Type III are microporous but with macroporous components, and type IV mesh are nonporous such as Silastic, Celligard, and Preclude [54, 55]. There lacks a clear recommendation on how to proceed with mesh exposure, especially for type I mesh. These cases add to the available literature regarding different types of mesh, their delayed complications, and treatment suggestions.

All data clearly shows that surgery is necessary when conservative measures fail, when there is high suspicion for severe osteitis, or when repeat mesh revisions are not successful. Surgery can occur via transvaginal excision, endoscopic assisted transvaginal excision, open laparotomy, or by minimally invasive intraperitoneal laparoscopic or robotic surgery. A literature review on the topic reveals no standard protocol for osteomyelitis related to POP-mesh [52, 56–58]. In February 2020, American Society of Obstetrics and Gynecology (ACOG) and International Urogynecological Association (IUGA) published a Joint Position to guide the management of mesh complications [57, 58]. Asymptomatic mesh exposure after SCP can be observed (Grade C recommendation) while understanding that three of four exposures will not resolve and may require surgery [57], which heals 93% of patients [59]. Similarly, Abbott et al. demonstrated that 60% of patients with mesh exposure need at least one surgical intervention to remove the mesh [60]. The 2019 National Institute for Health and Care Excellence recommends surgical intervention after 3 months of conservative management [57].

The patient of Case 1 underwent a trial of conservative management with antibiotics, however she required surgery once her clinical status acutely worsened. This patient became medically compromised, developed focal neurological deficits and her infection fistulised resulting in copious malodorous vaginal discharge leading to perineal excoriation.

Cases 2 and 3 presented patients requesting definitive surgical management after prior multiple failed mesh revisions attempts. Partial removal of mesh and the involved vaginal epithelium may be adequate for cases of limited vaginal exposure without pain (Grade D recommendation). However, office trimming with or without estrogen has a 75% risk of failure [18, 57, 61]. Repetitive trimming in the office is not recommended since it can distort the anatomy further (Grade D recommendation). According to the Joint Position, those who undergo surgical revision rather than office based trimming will still need additional surgery or complete excision in 37–50% of cases (Grace C recommendation). Focal vaginal pain without mesh exposure may require surgery if conservative measures are unsuccessful [57]. About 50% of patients undergoing mesh revision are successfully treated, but most require an abdominal surgery, and 25% require more than one surgery [57]. For persistent mesh-related pain, 50% of women with silicone mesh who attempt vaginal-specific repair ultimately need complete abdominal excision [57]. Cases 2 and 3 required complete intraperitoneal access removal of infected mesh after prior vaginal resection failures.

All above cases developed pelvic abscesses. Although there are reports of abscesses successfully managed by drainage alone (Grade C), these cases occurred within 14 days of SCP surgery [57]. Data is lacking for abscesses with delayed presentation, for which we recommend surgical intervention when conservative or partial-surgical interventions fail, or when severe symptoms persist. In those cases entire mesh must be removed. Similar to case 2 and 3 Unger et al. published a case of Gore-Tex soft tissue patch case that subsequently need complete removal after prior failed surgical attempts to partially remove it [24]. Our cases differ due to their prolonged interval from mesh placement to the time of osteitis. In these situations, surgeons should expect a chronically inflamed, distorted surgical field and must plan in advance to have different specialists equally involved and readily available.

In a patient with back pain and a history of SCP mesh, osteitis should be high on the differential given that 85% of SCP-osteitis cases present with back pain [62]. Physical exam with MRI of the lower spine is the gold standard for diagnosis [62]. Cultures can be helpful in directing targeted antibiotic therapy. Although some reported cases have responded to antibiotics alone (Grade I recommendation), most cases need multidisciplinary surgical team (Grade B recommendation), as this could be a life threatening condition [62]. The 2015 Infectious Disease Society of America (IDSA) recommend image-guided aspiration biopsy for patients with suspected vertebral osteomyelitis except when S. Aureus, S. Lugdunensis, or Brucella species are grown from blood cultures. However Jenson et al. recommends immediate empiric antibiotics to prevent infection along the spine [62]. Pathogens most commonly identified are staphylococcus and streptococcus, however fecal contamination may also be present in cases where a fistula is involved. Serratia Marcescens (SM) is a rod-shaped Gram-Negative facultative anaerobic, a rare bacterium that can cause osteomyelitis, particularly associated with IV recreational drug use or nosocomial infections [13]. SM fimbriae allow it to grasp onto surfaces, and its proteases enable it to thrive in anaerobic and aerobic environments [14]. Being intrinsically resistant to several beta-lactam antibiotics, first-line agents are instead Piperacillin-Tazobactam, a fluoroquinolone, an aminoglycoside, or a Carbapenem [14]. The regimen can then be tailored to susceptibility results. Given the nature and extent of infection, treatment requires 6–8 weeks of IV antibiotics, with most patients subsequently prescribed oral antibiotic therapy for a total duration of 12 weeks [8, 32, 63]. Case 2 demonstrates the aggressiveness of SM in the context of hospital-acquired infection, as it indolently grew and weakened the abdominal fascia causing incarcerated central hernia. This patient required a wound vacuum skin closure to allow repair sites to heal by secondary intention.

In presence of a severe infection, impaired mental capacity of elderly women may limit the ability to differentiate dementia from worsening sepsis. Individuals with history of POP mesh repairs with pain, abnormal vaginal discharge or bleeding discitis should have osteomyelitis high on the list of differentials and antibiotics should be initiated promptly if warranted. Consultation of FPMRS specialist familiar with above presentation along with physical exam and pelvic MRI helps for prompt diagnosis [53, 57]. Large mesh exposures, infection, severe symptoms, or involvement of bladder, bowel or bone require complete excision, understanding that complete removal of infected mesh from the posterior cul-de-sac in vicinity of the bladder and presacral space requires intra-abdominal access [57, 61]. Special attention must be paid to the bladder, ureters, rectum, and vagina, as well as the great pelvic vessels, particularly the left common iliac vein and its confluences or malformations. Although vaginal mesh complications have been well publicized, complications from intra-abdominal mesh placed by means of MIS for POP repair are limited. Compared to vaginally placed mesh, MIS intra-abdominal mesh is also more durable, however it carries its unique risks associated with general anesthesia, Trendelenburg positioning and pneumoperitoneum [42]. Otherwise, the unique risks are poorly published, with osteomyelitis only reported in several cases. There is limited guidance on how to approach an abdominal mesh complication. Expectant management can begin with antibiotics. Surgery is recommended if clinical status acutely worsens, symptoms are severe, if the patient has failed multiple attempts at mesh revision, or with new onset neurological deficits [18, 57, 61]. Although G. Willy Davila's report provides recommendations for managing small vs. large vaginal mesh exposures as well as its contractions and infection [50], Level I evidence are still lacking on how to manage infected mesh deep in the sacral region.

3. Conclusion

This case series presents an example of three patients who underwent open abdominal, laparoscopic and robotic POP repair several years prior, and subsequently developed mesh related osteomyelitis requiring complete removal of mesh. Of particular significance is the delayed onset of osteitis presenting up to a decade after mesh placement. This can be a challenge when patients are not the best historians either due to advanced age or other comorbidities. With an increased demand for POP prolapse surgeries as the population ages, mesh-related osteomyelitis will become more prevalent. Prospective randomized studies could help determine the ideal protocols for treatment of foreign body osteomyelitis. This short case series illustrates that mesh-related osteomyelitis after POP surgeries carries significant morbidity, its management can be technically challenging and should not be undertaken lightly. However it also demonstrates that mesh removal by means of MIS in the hands of an experienced surgical team utilizing DaVinci Robotic System is a good option and may be the preferred option among these challenging patients [52, 56].

Author details

Adriana Fulginiti[1], Frank Borao[2], Martin Michalewski[3]* and Robert A. Graebe[4]

1 Department of Obstetrics and Gynecology, Monmouth Medical Center, Long Branch, NJ, United States

2 Department of Bariatric Surgery, Monmouth Medical Center, Long Branch, NJ, United States

3 Department of Urogynecology, Monmouth Medical Center, Long Branch, NJ, United States

4 Department Chair of Obstetrics and Gynecology, Monmouth Medical Center, Long Branch, NJ, United States

*Address all correspondence to: michalewskimd@gmail.com

References

[1] Arthure, savage uterine prolapse and prolapse of the vaginal vault treated by sacral hysteropexy. The Journal of Obstetrics and Gynaecology of the British Empire. 1957;**64**:355-360

[2] Lane FE. Repair of post-hystectomy vaginal vault prolapse. Obstetrics & Gynecology. 1962;**20**:72-77

[3] Anger T, Mueller R, Tarnay R, et al. Robotic compared with laparoscopic Sacrocolpopexy: A randomized controlled trial. Obstetrics & Gynecology. 2014;**123**(1):5-12. DOI: 10.1097/AOG.0000000000000006

[4] Collins SA, Tulikangas PK, O'Sullivan DM. Effect of surgical approach on physical activity and pain control after sacral colpopexy. (Report). American Journal of Obstetrics and Gynecology. 2012;**206**(5):438.e1-438.e6

[5] Shepherd JP, Higdon HL 3rd, Stanford EJ, Mattox TF. Effect of suture selection on the rate of suture or mesh erosion and surgery failure in abdominal sacrocolpopexy. Female Pelvic Medicine & Reconstructive Surgery. 2010;**16**: 229-233

[6] Khan A, Alperin M, Wu N, et al. Comparative outcomes of open versus laparoscopic sacrocolpopexy among medicare beneficiaries. International Urogynecology Journal. 2013;**24**(11): 1883-1891. DOI: 10.1007/s00192-013-2088-9

[7] Callewaert G, Bosteels J, Housmans S, et al. Laparoscopic versus robotic-assisted sacrocolpopexy for pelvic organ prolapse: A systematic review. Gynecological Surgery. 2016;**13**(2):115-123. DOI: 10.1007/s10397-016-0930-z

[8] Weidner AC, Cundiff GW, Harris RL, Addison WA. Sacral osteomyelitis: An unusual complication of abdominal sacral colpopexy. Obstetrics and Gynecology. 1997; **90**(4 Pt 2):689-691. DOI: 10.1016/s0029-7844(97)00306-2

[9] Arbel R, Lavy Y. Vaginal vault prolapse: Choice of operation. Best Practice & Research Clinical Obstetrics & Gynaecology. 2005;**19**(6):959-977. DOI: 10.1016/j.bpobgyn.2005.08.011

[10] McDermott C, Park J, Terry C, Woodman P, Hale D. Laparoscopic sacral colpoperineopexy: Abdominal versus abdominal–vaginal posterior graft attachment. International Urogynecology Journal. 2011;**22**(4):469-475. DOI: 10.1007/s00192-010-1302-2

[11] Nezhat C. Laparoscopic sacral colpopexy for vaginal vault prolapse. Obstetrics and Gynecology. 1994;**84**:885-888

[12] Di Marco DS, Chow GK, Gettman MT, Elliott DS. Robotic-assisted laparoscopic sacrocolpopexy for treatment of vaginal vault prolapse. Urology (Ridgewood, NJ). 2004;**63**(2): 373-376. DOI: 10.1016/j.urology.2003.09.033

[13] Marco D, Chow, Gettman, et al. Robotic-assisted laparoscopic sacrocolpopexy for treatment of vaginal vault prolapse. Urology. 2004;**63**:373

[14] Geller EJ, Siddiqui NY, Wu JM, Visco AG. Short-term outcomes of robotic sacrocolpopexy compared with abdominal sacrocolpopexy. Obstetrics and Gynecology. 2008;**112**(6): 1201-1206. DOI: 10.1097/AOG.0b013e31818ce394

[15] Margulies RU, Lewicky-Gaupp C, Fenner DE, et al. Complications requiring reoperation following vaginal mesh kit procedures for prolapse. American Journal of Obstetrics and Gynecology. 2008;**199**(678):e1-e4

[16] Mowat A, Maher C, Ballard E. Surgical outcomes for low-volume vs high-volume surgeons in gynecology surgery: A systematic review and meta-analysis. American Journal of Obstetrics and Gynecology. 2016;**215**(1):21-33. DOI: 10.1016/j.ajog.2016.02.048

[17] Toomey P, Teta A, Patel K, Ross S, Rosemurgy A. High-volume surgeons vs high-volume hospitals: Are best outcomes more due to who or where? The American Journal of Surgery. 2016;**211**(1):59-63. DOI: 10.1016/j.amjsurg.2015.08.021

[18] Bergersen A, Hinkel C, Funk J, Twiss CO. Management of vaginal mesh exposure: A systematic review. Arab Journal of Urology. 2019;**17**(1):40-48. DOI: 10.1080/2090598X.2019.1589787

[19] Update on the Safety and Effectiveness of Transvaginal Placement for Pelvic Organ Prolapse, July 2011 [Internet]. U.S. Food and Drug Administration; 2020. Available from: https://www.fda.gov/media/81123/download

[20] Barbalat Y, Tunuguntla H. Surgery for pelvic organ prolapse: A historical perspective. Current Urology Reports. 2012;**13**(3):256-261. DOI: 10.1007/s11934-012-0249-x

[21] Ortman J, Velkoff A. An Aging Nation: The Older Population in the United States. Washington, D.C: U.S. Department of Commerce, Economics and Statistics Administration, U.S. Census Bureau; 2014. Available from: https://www.census.gov/library/publications/2014/demo/p25-1140.html

[22] Kirby A, Luber K, Menefee S. An update on the current and future demand for care of pelvic floor disorders in the United States. American Journal of Obstetrics and Gynecology. 2013;**209**(6):584.e1-584.e5. DOI: 10.1016/j.ajog.2013.09.011

[23] Wu JM, Hundley AF, Fulton RG, Myers ER. Forecasting the prevalence of pelvic floor disorders in U.S. women: 2010 to 2050. Obstetrics and Gynecology. 2009;**114**(6):1278-1283

[24] FDA Orders Makers of Women's Surgical Mesh to Stop Selling the Products. Dow Jones Institutional News. 2019. Available from: http://search.proquest.com/docview/2210255794/

[25] Gornall J. Vaginal mesh implants: Putting the relations between UK doctors and industry in plain sight. BMJ: British Medical Journal (Online). 2018;**363**. DOI: 10.1136/bmj.k4164

[26] Roovers JP. Collaboration with the mesh industry: Who needs who? International Urogynecology Journal. 2016;**27**(9):1293-1295. DOI: 10.1007/s00192-016-3075-8. Epub 2016 Jul 13

[27] Sung VW, Rogers RG, Schaffer JI, Balk EM, Uhlig K, Lau J, et al. Graft use in transvaginal pelvic organ prolapse repair: A systematic review. Obstetrics & Gynecology. 2008;**112**(5):1131-1142. DOI: 10.1097/AOG.0b013e3181898ba9

[28] Abed et al. Incidence and management of graft erosion, wound granulation, and dyspareunia following vaginal prolapse repair with graft materials: A systematic review. International Urogynecology Journal. 2011;**22**(7):789-798

[29] Caquant F, Collinet P, Debodinance P, Berrocal J, Garbin O, Rosenthal C, et al. Safety of trans vaginal mesh procedure: Retrospective study of 684 patients. The Journal of Obstetrics and Gynaecology Research. 2008;**34**(4):449-456. DOI: 10.1111/j.1447-0756.2008.00820.x

[30] Aungst MJ, Friedman EB, von Pechmann WS, Horbach NS, Welgoss JA. De novo stress incontinence and pelvic muscle symptoms after

transvaginal mesh repair. American Journal of Obstetrics and Gynecology. 2009;**201**(1):73.e1-73.e7. DOI: 10.1016/j.ajog.2009.02.028. Epub 2009 Apr 23

[31] Rabin RC. Trial of Synthetic Mesh in Pelvic Surgery Ends Early. The New York Times; 2010. Available from: http://www.nytimes.com/2010/ 10/26/health/research/26complications.html?_r=0

[32] The Royal Australian and New Zealand College of Obstetricians and Gynaecologists. Polypropylene Vaginal Mesh Implants for Vaginal Prolapse. Renewed November 2016. Available from: www.ranzcog.edu.au/getattachment/Statements-Guidelines/Gynaecology/Polypropylene-Vaginal-Mesh-Implants-for-Vaginal-Pr/Polypropylene-vaginal-mesh-implants-for-vaginal-prolapse-(C-Gyn-20)-Review-November-2016.pdf?lang=en-AU&ext=.pdf

[33] Meier BFDA. Orders Surgical Mesh Makers to Study Risks. The New York Times; 2012. Available from: http://www.nytimes.com/2012/01/05/health/research/fda-orders-more-study-on-surgical-mesh-risks.html [Accessed: December 31, 2012]

[34] Consumer Reports Magazine Staff. Dangerous devices: Most medical implants have never been tested for safety. Consumer Reports. 2012:24Y29

[35] Wu Y, Welk B. Revisiting current treatment options for stress urinary incontinence and pelvic organ prolapse: A contemporary literature review. Research and Reports in Urology. 2019;**11**:179-188. Available from: https://doaj.org/article/85f77c35fd9c436fb6c15cfae9e27e56

[36] Cornella J. Management of stress urinary incontinence. Reviews in Urology. 2004;**6**(Suppl. 5):S18-S25

[37] Douseki T, Tanaka A. Self-powered wireless disposable sensor for welfare application. Annual International Conference of the IEEE Engineering in Medicine and Biology Society. 2013;**2013**:1664-1667. DOI: 10.1109/EMBC.2013.6609837

[38] Wright T. Adult Incontinence Market is Baby Booming. Nonwovens Industry. 2013. Available from: https://www.nonwovens-industry.com/the-ai-market-is-baby-booming

[39] Barber MD, Brubaker L, Burgio KL, et al. Comparison of 2 transvaginal surgical approaches and perioperative behavioral therapy for apical vaginal prolapse: The OPTIMAL randomized trial. Journal of the American Medical Association. 2014;**311**(10):1023-1034. DOI: 10.1001/jama.2014.1719

[40] Muffly TM, Diwadkar GB, Paraiso MF. Lumbosacral osteomyelitis after robot-assisted total laparoscopic hysterectomy and sacral colpopexy. International Urogynecology Journal. 2010;**21**(12):1569-1571. DOI: 10.1007/s00192-010-1187-0. Epub 2010 Jun 8

[41] Hart SR, Weiser EB, Hart SR, Weiser EB. Abdominal sacral colpopexy mesh erosion resulting in a sinus tract formation and sacral abscess. Obstetrics and Gynecology. 2004;**103**:1037-1040

[42] Linder B, Elliott D. Robotic Sacrocolpopexy: How does it compare with other prolapse repair techniques? Current Urology Reports. 2013;**14**(3):235-239. DOI: 10.1007/s11934-012-0299-0

[43] Cho E, Um M, Kim S, Jung H. A study on laparoscopic sacral colpopexy for uterine prolapse. Journal of Menopausal Medicine. 2017;**23**(3):190-195. DOI: 10.6118/jmm.2017.23.3.190

[44] Mattimore J, Cheetham P, Katz A. The history of pelvic organ prolapse from antiquity to present day. Journal of Urology. 2015;**193**(4):E590-E591

[45] Crosby EC, Abernethy M, Berger MB, et al. Symptom resolution after operative management of complications from transvaginal mesh. Obstetrics and Gynecology. 2014;**123**:134-139

[46] Deval B, Fauconnier A, Repiquet D, Liou Y, Montuclard B, Fritel X, et al. Traitement chirurgical des prolapsus génito-urinaires par voie abdominale. A propos d'une série de 232 cas [Surgical treatment of genitourinary prolapse by the abdominal approach. Apropos of a series of 232 cases]. Annales de Chirurgie. 1997;**51**(3):256-265

[47] Daneshgari F, Hijaz A, Moore C, Aleman M, Kaouk J. Robotic laparoscopic sacrocolpopexy with or without uteropexy. Journal of Urology. 2005;**173**(4):136-136

[48] Munz Y, Moorthy K, Kudchadkar R, Hernandez J, Martin S, Darzi A, et al. Robotic assisted rectopexy. The American Journal of Surgery. 2004;**187**(1):88-92. DOI: 10.1016/j.amjsurg.2002.11.001

[49] Banerjie C, Noe K. Laparoscopic pectopexy: A new technique of prolapse surgery for obese patients. Archives of Gynecology and Obstetrics. 2011;**284**(3):631-635. DOI: 10.01107/s00404-010-1687-7

[50] Smith A, Davila G. Take this simplified approach to correcting exposure of vaginal mesh: By proceeding stepwise, uncomplicated exposures lend themselves to the generalist's care. Here are management pearls, cautions, and gauges of success (Surgical Techniques) (case study). OBG Management. 2011;**23**(7):29-40

[51] Maher C, Feiner B, Baessler K, et al. Surgical management of pelvic organ prolapse in women. Cochrane Database of Systematic Reviews. 2010;**4**:CD004014

[52] Chamsy D, Lee T, Chamsy D. Laparoscopic excision of sacrocolpopexy mesh. Journal of Minimally Invasive Gynecology. 2014;**21**(6):986-986. DOI: 10.1016/j.jmig.2014.07.011

[53] Müller P, Berchtold C, Kuemmerli C, Ruzza C, Z'Graggen K, Steinemann D. Spondylodiscitis after minimally invasive recto- and colpo-sacropexy: Report of a case and systematic review of the literature. Journal of Minimal Access Surgery. 2020;**16**(1):5-12. DOI: 10.4103/jmas.JMAS_235_18

[54] Amid P. Classification of biomaterials and their relative complications in an abdominal wall hernia surgery. Hernia. 1997;**1**:15-21. DOI: 10.1007/BF02426382

[55] Zambon J, Badlani G. Vaginal mesh exposure presentation, evaluation, and management. Current Urology Reports. 2016;**17**(9):1-8. DOI: 10.1007/s11934-016-0617-z

[56] Heisler CA, Casiano ER, Klingele CJ, Gebhart JB, Trabuco EC. Ureteral injury during vaginal mesh excision: Role of prevention and treatment options. American Journal of Obstetrics and Gynecology. 2012;**207**(6):e3-e4. DOI: 10.1016/j.ajog.2012.09.010

[57] Rardin C, Duckett J, Milani A, Paván L, Rogo-Gupta L, Twiss C. Joint position statement on the management of mesh-related complications for the FPMRS specialist. International Urogynecology Journal. 2020;**31**(4):679-694. DOI: 10.1007/s00192-020-04248-x

[58] Management of mesh and graft complications in gynecologic surgery. Obstetrics and Gynecology. 2017;**129**(4): E102-E108

[59] Skoczylas L, Shepherd J, Smith K, Lowder J. Managing mesh exposure following vaginal prolapse repair: A decision analysis comparing conservative versus surgical treatment.

International Urogynecology Journal. 2013;**24**(1):119-125. DOI: 10.1007/s00192-012-1847-3

[60] Abbott S, Unger CA, Evans JM, et al. Evaluation and management of complications from synthetic mesh after pelvic reconstructive surgery: A multicenter study. American Journal of Obstetrics and Gynecology. 2014;**210**:163.e1-163.e8

[61] Urinary incontinence and pelvic organ prolapse in women: Management. NICE guideline. National Institute for Health and Care Excellence. 2019. Available from: www.nice.org.uk/guidance/ng123/resources/urinary-incontinence-and-pelvic-organ-prolapse-in-women-management-pdf-66141657205189 [Accessed: April 22, 2019]

[62] Spelzini F, Frigerio M, Manodoro S, Interdonato M, Cesana M, Verri D, et al. Modified McCall coldoplasty versus Shull suspension in pelvic prolapse primary repair: A retrospective study. International Urogynecology Journal. 2017;**28**(1):65-71. DOI: 10.1007/s00192-016-3016-6

[63] Jenson MDAV, Scranton R, Antosh DD, Simpson RK. Lumbosacral osteomyelitis and discitis with Phlegmon following laparoscopic sacral colpopexy. Cureus. 2016;**8**(7):e671. DOI: 10.7759/cureus.671. Erratum in: Cureus. 2016;**8**(10):c5

Chapter 3

Perspective Chapter: Total Vaginal Hysterectomy for Unprolapsed Uterus

Petre Bratila

Abstract

Vaginal hysterectomy was the first method to extract the uterus. Vaginal hysterectomy goes back a long way into the history of medicine. Although the first hysterectomy was carried out by Themison of Athens in the year 20 B.C., the idea of extracting the uterus through the vagina was first mentioned in 120 B.C. by Soranus of Ephesos, a distinguished obstetrician. *The first elective vaginal hysterectomy* was performed by J. Conrad Langenbeck in 1813. The patient was a 50-year-old multipara, who suffered from chronic pelvic pain attributed to a prolapsed uterus with a hard, bleeding tumor. The operation was carried out in challenging conditions, without anesthesia, proper instruments, or surgical assistants. Until the early 1950s, vaginal hysterectomy was the method of choice for removing the uterus. With the widespread introduction of general anesthesia and antibiotic therapy, the site of vaginal hysterectomy was taken over by abdominal hysterectomy. With the introduction of minimally invasive surgery in gynecology, vaginal hysterectomy has regained its place. Harry Reich performed the first total laparoscopic hysterectomy in 1989, being one of the most renowned vaginal surgeons, and he still claims at the beginning of the 21st century that ... *when the first choice of approach for hysterectomy is possible, is the vaginal route*. This chapter presents the relevant anatomy from the point of view of the vaginal surgeon and the standard technique used by the author in over 5,000 vaginal hysterectomies. All intraoperative drawings and photographs are original.

Keywords: pelvic anatomy, vaginal hysterectomy, surgical technique

1. Introduction

1.1 The uterus

The uterus is an organ with a particular anatomic situation localized with the uterine body intraperitoneally, the isthmus extra-peritoneally, and the cervix can be considered visible intravaginal organs. The uterine body is coated by the visceral peritoneum, which intimately adheres to its sides. In front, the visceral peritoneum reflects it on the bladder and in the back to the rectum. On the lateral side, the visceral uterine peritoneum detaches from the two sides of the uterus into two sheets that are joined to each other but are anatomically distinct and surgically separable, forming *broad ligaments*.

The uterus is maintained in anatomical position inside the pelvis by two systems: a *suspension and orientation system* for its intra-abdominal part and by a *supporting system* for the retroperitoneally part of the isthmus, cervix, and upper vagina. (Yabuky).

2. The suspension and orientation system of the uterus

The suspension and orientation system of the uterus consists of *broad ligaments, round ligaments*, *infundibulopelvic ligaments,* and the *parietal peritoneum*.

Round ligaments play a minor supporting role, the main one being the orientation of the uterus. Round ligaments are active elements that contain an essential contingent of smooth muscle fibers. The anatomic origin is located cranially at the level of the uterine fundus, under the insertion of uterine tubes. Each round ligament engages through the homologous inguinal canal, to be inserted into the thickness of the labia majora.

Broad ligaments result in the lateral reflection of the pelvic parietal peritoneum on each side to the two sides of the uterus. After the peritoneal sheets detach from the pelvic walls, they re-join and form two peritoneal folds cranially suspended by the round ligaments. Frontally, broad ligaments are trapezoidal, with a caudally located base. The orientation of the plan containing the broad ligaments depends on the position of the uterus (ante- or retroversion).

The *pelvic parietal peritoneum* is an essential support for the uterine body, which becomes visible, particularly in vaginal hysterectomy. Access to the superior connective-vascular pedicle (round ligament, utero-ovarian ligament, and superior uterine pedicle) is profoundly difficult if the peritoneum of the broad ligaments is not sectioned as far as possible so that it loses contact with the pelvic parietal and visceral peritoneum. The tensile strength of the peritoneum and the perforation strength of broad ligaments are outstanding. Even if the uterus is disconnected from its primary support, it is held in the pelvis by the peritoneal connections.

Infundibulopelvic ligaments indirectly suspend the uterus via the ovary and utero-ovarian ligaments. Infundibulo pelvic ligaments have a mesenteric structure with a vascular and nerve fiber content that generally does not exert a suspension tension on the uterus. In pathological situations that cause their shortening and retraction generates resistance to the tendency to caudal traction of the uterus.

3. The supporting system of the uterus

The supporting system reunites all the elements that work together to maintain the uterus in its intrapelvic anatomical position and resist the descending tendency generated by the weight of the intestines at rest or under effort.

Biomechanical studies show that the support of the uterus and the upper part of the vagina are provided by the *four-wire system*, where the *cardinal ligaments* anchor the pericervical ring vertically and *uterosacral ligaments* dorsally.

The supporting system anchors the uterus and vagina to the pelvic brim: the *pubocervical ligaments* anteriorly and the *transverse cervical ligament (cardinal ligaments)* cranially and *uterosacral ligament* posteriorly. All these ligaments converge to the pericervical ring. The pericervical ring of the uterus is the insertion area for the supporting structures, and it forms a virtual delimitation between the intraperitoneal and extraperitoneal parts of the uterus. Pericervical ring also offers support for a vaginal vault.

Transverse cervical ligaments (cardinal ligaments) are oriented vertically. They are formed by two segments: a fibroconnective structure that joins the uterosacral ligaments close to the pericervical ring and a mesenteric structure containing blood, lymphatic vessels, and nerves as a distal segment. In the cardinal ligament, the deep uterine vein delimits a cranial segment containing vessels and a caudal one containing nerves (**Figure 1**).

Cardinal ligaments provide reliable support for the vascular and lymphatic axes that converge or emerge in the uterus. Their fibers dissipate in the

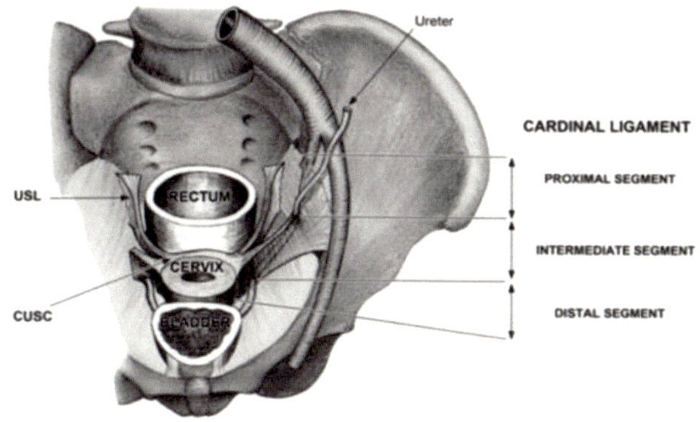

Figure 1.
The cardinal ligament consists of three segments: Proximal and intermediate segments containing the mesenteric elements and the terminal ureter and a common segment with the homologous uterosacral ligament, which is the main support element of the pericervical ring.

pubocervicovesical fascia towards the cervix uteri and superior vagina at the level of the cervical ring, and the fascial and areolar structures towards the pelvic walls, structures that cover the pelvic diaphragm, the obturator pelvic fascia, and the tendinous arch of the pelvis (arcus taendineus fascia pelvis-ATFP). (Campbell).

The sacrouterine ligaments have their origin in the posterior part of the pericervical ring and the posterior-lateral portion of the vaginal fornices, structures that continue the cardinal ligaments. Posteriorly, the uterosacral ligaments insert into the presacral fascia at the level of the sacroiliac joints S2-S4. Utero-sacral ligaments run in the supra levator part of the vagina, forming with the infra levator segment at an angle of 130°. (Chen) (**Figure 2**).

Like the cardinal ligaments, the uterosacral ligaments defined three segments: a proximal segment that merges with the cardinal ligament, an intermediate segment that represents the structure that can be used as a suspension element, and a distal segment that merges with the presacral fascia. Sacrouterine ligaments contain nervous

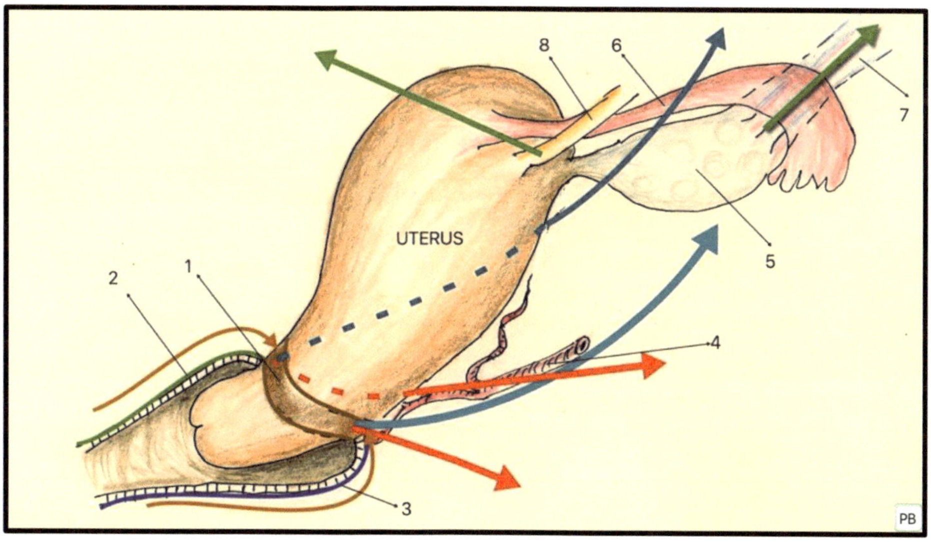

Figure 2.
Orienting-supporting *system of the uterus* supporting system*: 1 = pericervical ring. Spatial orientation of the cardinal (blue arrow) and uterosacral ligaments (red arrow): 4 = uterine artery 5 = ovary, 6 = fallopian tube, 2 = pubocervical fascia, 3 = rectovaginal septum.* Orienting system *(green arrow): 8 = round ligament, 7 = infundibulo-pelvic ligament.*

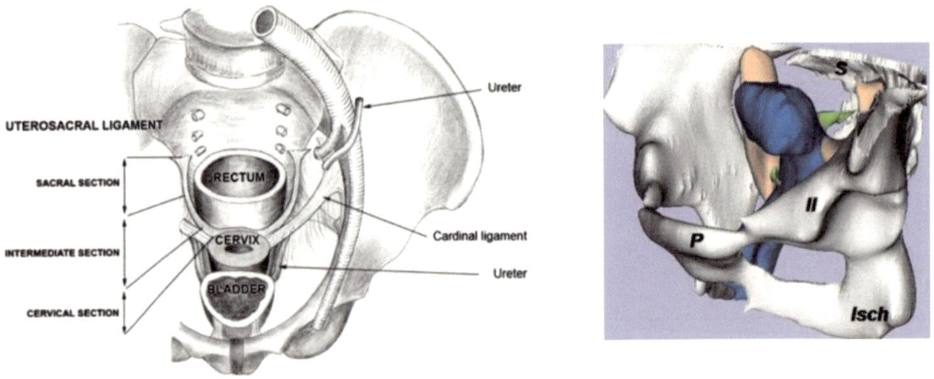

Figure 3.
Definition of three segments of uterosacral ligaments. MRI reconstruction -spatial disposition of posteriorly oriented uterosacral ligaments (in green) and cardinal ligaments oriented vertically (in beige yellow), P = pubis arch, Isch = ischion, Il = ilion, S = sacrum.

fibers from the superior hypogastric plexus. Those innervating the urinary bladder are of particular importance in nerve-sparing surgery for cervical cancer (**Figure 3**).

4. The connective-vascular pedicles of the uterus

Vaginal hysterectomy consists of disconnection from below of all elements that maintain the uterus in anatomical position.

From the vaginal point of view, the uterus suspension-supporting system consists of three main connective-vascular pedicles; lower, middle, and upper pedicles.

like abdominal hysterectomy, where the lower pedicle is most difficult to approach, vaginal hysterectomy solves this operative step as the first maneuver of the disconnection of the uterus.

a. Lower Pedicle

On the caudal side, the cervix and uterine isthmus provide insertion for two fibrous-connective structures: anteriorly, *the vesicouterine ligaments* (bladder pillars), and posteriorly, the *uterosacral ligaments*. In the sagittal plane, the two ligaments are located approximately at the same level. When the uterus is not prolapsed, it can be treated as a single pedicle with an anterior division and a posterior one, the superior vagina remaining anchored even after its disconnection. The natural connections of these pedicles with the superior vagina must be preserved regardless of the hysterectomy method because this is the most efficient method to prevent post-hysterectomy vaginal vault prolapse.

The vesicouterine ligaments join the bladder walls with the anterolateral edges of the cervix. During the vaginal hysterectomy, the bladder pillars can be visualized by cranial retraction of the bladder with a Breisky-Navratil retractor after the *cervicovesical ligament* has been sectioned and the bladder has been detached from the cervix, opening the vesicouterine space.

The juxta vesical ureter, surrounded by fatty tissue, is located in the thickness of each pillar. The *vesicouterine* ligaments have a medial and a lateral part. To be able to release the ureter, the two parts must be sectioned at the level of their cervical insertion. The vesicouterine ligaments contain the superior vascular-nervous pedicles of the urinary bladder.

The *uterosacral ligaments* are the most robust structures supporting the uterus. The confluence of the uterosacral ligaments on the uterus forms a small depression known as the *torus uterinus,* always situated at the level of uterine isthmus regardless of the length of the cervix. Torus uterinus marks the area where the visceral uterine peritoneum conjoins with the rectum at the level of the pouch of Douglas. Before the opening of the rectouterine peritoneal fold, we will see a variable amount of fatty tissue, which forms the *yellow line* that announces to the surgeon the dissection layer and the imminent appearance of the underlying rectum. *The fat belongs to the rectum and not to the vaginal wall.*

The uterosacral ligaments on the lateral sides, towards their sacral insertion, are flanked by the hypogastric nerve, which, along with the pelvic nerves, will be part of the inferior hypogastric plexus. For this reason, sectioning the uterosacral ligaments in radical vaginal hysterectomy as close as possible to the sacral insertion bears the risk of urinary disorders occurring through bladder denervation. Laterally and caudally, the uterosacral ligaments continue with the superior paracolpium, and a division of them achieves the upper level of suspension of the vagina (Delancey).

Campbell identified three distinct histologic regions of the uterosacral ligament. At the cervical attachment, the ligament was made up of carefully packed bundles of smooth muscle, abundant medium-sized and small blood vessels, and small nerve bundles. The intermediate third of the ligament was composed of predominantly connective tissue and only a few scattered smooth muscle fibers, nerve elements, and blood vessels. The sacral third was almost entirely composed of loose strands of connective tissue and intermingled fat, few vessels, nerves, and lymphatics.

The mechanical strength of the uterosacral ligaments is remarkable. The cervical and intermediate portions of the uterosacral ligament supported more than 17 kg of weight before failure. (Nichols) (**Figure 4**).

b. Middle Pedicle

The middle connective-vascular pedicle consists of the cardinal ligaments and a variable contingent of fibers that are part of the uterosacral ligaments. Vaginally, each cardinal ligament has a fibrous-connective segment consisting of inferior fibers of the uterosacral ligament and a cranially located vascular segment, which consists of the superior bundle of the cardinal ligament and uterine vascular pedicle. The two segments can be surgically treated as a single pedicle or as separate depending on the thickness and insertion area of the uterine edge (Shiff).

On its cranial aspect, the cardinal ligament is crossed by the ureter under the crossing-point with the uterine artery. The distance between the lateral side of the cervix and isthmus and the wall of the pelvis is approximately 4–5 cm. The ureter crosses the cardinal ligament halfway, approximately 2–2.5 cm from the cervix. The ureteral risk is reduced in vaginal hysterectomy because, once the lower pedicle is cut, the cardinal ligament is elongated, removing the ureter from the operator's field. (Kovak) (**Figure 5**).

c. Upper Pedicle

The upper pedicle consists of *round ligaments*, *uterine tubes*, and *utero-ovarian ligaments*. The tubes and ovaries are indirectly supported by the *infundibulopelvic ligament*, which offers support to the pelvic wall. The upper

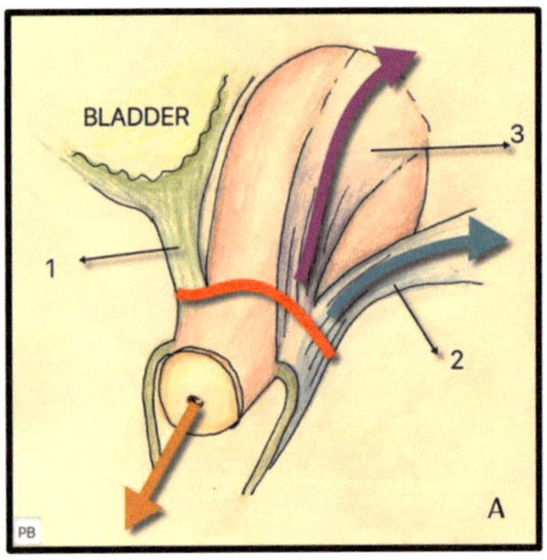

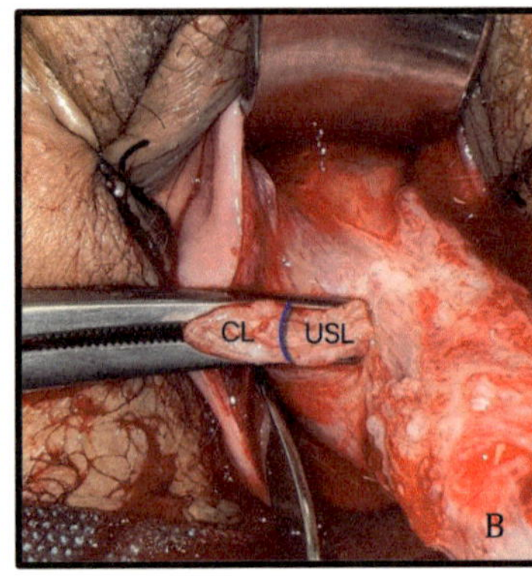

Figure 4.
A. Lower connective-vascular pedicle (cardinal uterosacral complex -CUSC the first pedicle in vaginal hysterectomy). 1 = cervicovesical ligament, 2 = uterosacral ligaments, 3 = cardinal ligament. Redline mark where the same pedicle might secure bladder pillar, uterosacral ligaments, and cardinal ligaments. B. Lower connective pedicle at vaginal hysterectomy with distinct uterosacral ligament (USL) and cardinal ligament (CL) in the same pedicle.

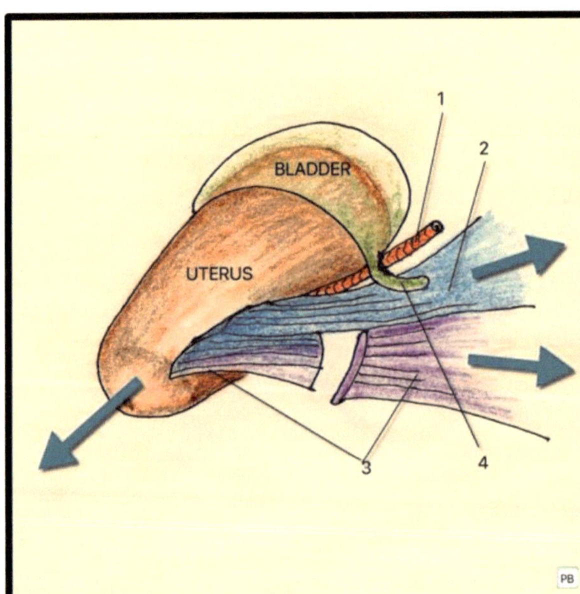

Figure 5.
Middle pedicle. 1 = uterine artery, 2 = cardinal ligament, 3 = inferior pedicle cut, 4 = parametrial ureter. Once cut, the uterosacral ligament's traction on the cervix makes the cardinal ligament elongated and removes the ureter from the surgical field.

pedicle, which does not have a significant supporting role, maintains the uterus in anatomical position and stands against the force that tends to push it through the pelvic opening. During the vaginal hysterectomy, the upper pedicle is the most problematic one in terms of strategy regarding the extraction of the uterus from the pelvic cavity.

The primary vascular element of the upper pedicle is the *Tubo ovarian arch*, contained in the thickness of the *mesosalpinx*. The infundibulopelvic pedicle becomes the main vascular element when an adnexectomy is an option. The resistance of the superior pedicle to traction is due to the intrinsic elasticity of the connective elements in the ligament structures and the resistance of the leaf of broad ligaments. Chronic inflammatory processes may cause the adhesion of ovaries to the posterior leaf of broad ligament or parietal peritoneum of fossa ovaries, which leads to the fixation of the adnexa to the walls of the pelvis. Vaginal adnexectomy is difficult in these cases.

5. Uterine blood supply

The uterus is a highly vascular organ with two arterial and two venous systems intertwined.

The primary arterial system is composed of the *uterine* and *vaginal arteries*, which originate from the hypogastric artery. *The ovarian arteries*, which originate from the aorta on each side and the *funicular artery*, from the external iliac artery, form the second arterial system. The two systems communicate through *utero-ovarian anastomotic* vessels.

Between the *uterine artery* and the *vaginal artery*, there are many anastomotic branches, and simple occlusion of the uterine and ovarian artery is not enough to stop blood flow in the uterine body.

The venous system is composed of the *uterine veins* (superficial and deep), which drain the blood in the *hypogastric veins* on each side, and *the ovarian veins* which drain on the right side into the vena cava inferior and on the left side into the left renal vein.

5.1 Arterial blood supply

The arterial blood supply is provided by three different sources: the *uterine artery*, the *utero-ovarian artery,* and the *vaginal arteries.*

a. *The uterine artery* is the primary blood supply source for a uterus in a reasonable condition. During pregnancy, the utero-ovarian artery becomes the second significant source, doubling its diameter. In non-pregnant women, the diameter of the left uterine artery is 1.6 mm, and for the right artery, it is 1.4 mm. The diameter of the uterine artery may vary for large uteri, up to 5 mm.

The origin of the uterine artery can be encountered most often in a common trunk with the umbilical artery, which arises as to the terminal branch from the previous division of the hypogastric artery. However, there is also the anatomic variant of direct origin from the hypogastric artery. From its origin, the uterine artery follows a 3–5 cm intrapelvic trajectory, approaching the cervix at a constant distance of approximately 2–2.5 cm without coming into contact.

The level where the uterine artery enters the uterine body, regardless of the shape or size of the uterus, corresponds to the level of the internal cervical orifice (**Figure 6**).

In its trajectory, the uterine artery has three distinct segments: *a parietal segment*, a *transversal one*, and a *lateral-uterine* one.

In the *parietal segment*, the uterine artery is in contact with the pelvic wall and is located on the side of the ureter, which crosses it in places, underneath and medially. In this segment, the artery is rectilinear and is accompanied by the uterine veins, which can be injured during maneuvers to identify its original ligation.

The *transversal segment* or (intra-parametrial segment) of the uterine artery is approximately 3 cm long. In this segment, the artery has the most important relation to the ureter, which is located outside of it. There is a cleavage space between

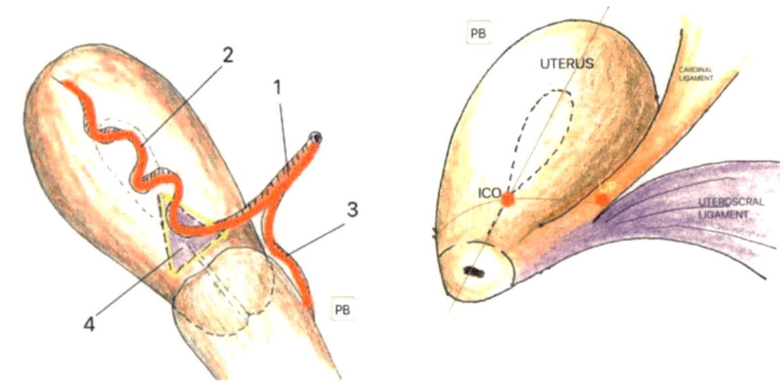

Figure 6.
The point where the uterine artery reaches the uterus is constant at the level of the internal cervical orifice. ICO = internal cervical orifice, UP = uterine point. 1 = main uterine artery, 2 = ascending branch of the uterine artery, three = descending branches of the uterine artery. 4 = Beliaeva triangle.

the ureter and the artery. At this level, the uterine artery emits a nutritional branch for the corresponding ureteral segment. During maneuvers to release the uterus in case of radical hysterectomy, this branch "holds" the ureter in the surgeon's attempt to move it caudally. The ligation or coagulation of this vessel is necessary because subserosa ureteral hematoma may appear, which can compromise the viability of the ureter on this segment.

The uterine artery reaches the uterus in a triangular zone near the isthmus (Beliaeva triangle) situated at the base of the broad ligaments at three o clock for the right side and nine o clock for the left side (from the vaginal point of view). The descending uterine artery supplies the isthmus, cervix, and upper vagina. The ascending uterine artery supplies the body of the uterus. The ascending uterine artery is tortuous and gives rise to 10–12 arcuate arteries that course between the outer and middle thirds of the myometrium.

The crossing point of the uterine artery with the ureter is located sideways, approximately 20 mm away from the cervix and 10–12 mm cranially from the lateral vaginal fornix. At this level, there are two venous currents, one in front and another in the back of the ureter, which is predisposed to bleed during maneuvers to unroof the parametrial ureter (**Figure** 7).

The *lateral-uterine segment* of the uterine artery starts from the crossing point and emits an *ascending branch* that borders the whole uterine edge up to the horn, as well as a *descending branch*, from which the cervicovaginal (superior vaginal branch) arteries arise. The ascending branch is tortuous and intimately adhered to the uterine edge-front-side and is accompanied by the uterine veins.

Between the right and left sides of the uterine body, the arcuate arteries are anastomosed by collateral and small, direct branches. At the uterine fundus, approximately 15 mm away from the insertion of the tube, the ascending uterine artery divides into two branches: *the fundic artery*, which supplies the fundus of the uterus on each side, and the *internal tubal artery*, which is routed under the utero-ovarian ligament, into the mesosalpinx.

a. *The ovarian artery* included in the *infundibulopelvic* ligament, after crossing the external iliac artery and vein, emits two branches, a tubal and an ovarian one, which is anastomosed between them by short arteries. The uterine artery provides the primary blood flow, but in particular conditions, such as after uterine embolization or in pregnancy, more than 80% of blood flow can be provided by the ovarian artery.

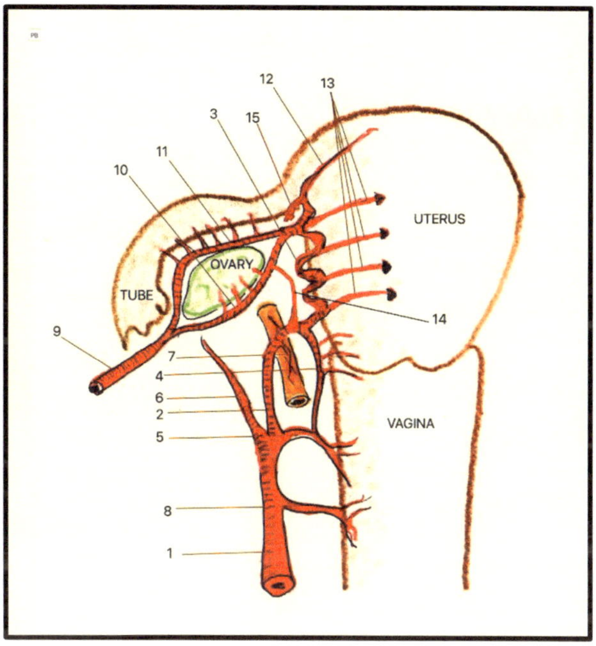

Figure 7.
Arterial supply of uterus and vagina. 1 = arterial trunk of hypogastric artery, 2 = Main trunk of the uterine artery, 3 = the ascending branch of the uterine artery, 4 = the descending branch of uterine artery (superior vaginal artery), five = inferior vaginal artery, 6 = umbilical vesical artery, 7 = ureteral branches from the uterine artery, 8 = middle hemorrhoidal artery, nine = ovarian artery, ten = ovarian arch between ovarian and uterine branches, 11 = tubal arch between ovarian and uterine branches, 12 = fundal branch of the uterine artery, 13 = arcuate arteries from right side, 14 = anastomotic branch between the uterine artery and ovarian arch, 15 = funicular branch (round ligament) artery.

b. *Vaginal arteries*, in more than 90% of cases, have their origin in the descending branch of the uterine artery, but they may also come directly from the hypogastric artery. Arterial blood flow of the vagina has three primary sources:

- A branch from the uterine artery.
- The vaginal artery.
- The middle hemorrhoidal artery.

The source of the uterine artery is composed of vesicovaginal and cervicovaginal branches and ensures the blood flow for the upper part of the vagina. The correct vaginal artery (lower vaginal artery or large vaginal artery) originates from the hypogastric artery. The artery from both sides anastomose in the midline and forms the longitudinal artery from the cervix to the vulva named the *azygos artery of the vagina*. The hemorrhoidal artery emits some branches for the posterior side of the vagina.

a. The *funicular artery* (artery of the round ligament) is an auxiliary blood supply source that can become a significant source in case of bilateral ligation or embolization of the hypogastric artery.

b. The *anastomotic branch* between the ovarian and ascending branches of the uterine artery can be found in broad ligaments.

The bilateral ligature of the anterior trunk of hypogastric arteries cannot stop the blood flow into the pelvis. Two primary sources ensure arterial collateral circulation of the pelvis:

Branches of the hypogastric artery

- Iliolumbar arteries
- Lateral sacral arteries
- Middle hemorrhoidal arteries

Systemic circulation

- Lumbar arteries
- Middle sacral artery
- Superior hemorrhoidal arteries

5.2 Venous blood supply

Venous blood from the uterine body comes from the veins located in the thickness of the myometrium, which is venous sinuses with reduced endothelial cover. Venous blood drains into two collecting veins on each side of the uterus, with anastomoses in between. The collateral venous blood supply is significant concerning the alternative route for blood flow in case of significant obstruction of main venous branches.

Collateral venous circulation of the uterus can be done in three main ways:

- The *veins of the round ligament* drain into the superficial epigastric vein and femoral vein.
- The *utero-ovarian veins* are arranged in an anterior plane in the mesosalpinx and in a posterior plane that is a satellite of the utero-ovarian ligament. On the external extremity of the broad ligament, these two venous networks are anastomosed, forming the *pampiniform plexus* that is part of the constitution of *infundibulopelvic* ligaments. These plexuses go up through the lumbar region and drain into the inferior vena cava on the right and into the left renal vein on the left.
- The *uterovaginal veins* are organized in two planes, a preureteral one and a retroureteral one, which is anastomosed with the perivesical, perivaginal plexus and drain into the hypogastric veins.

The venous blood supply of the vagina consists of veins that come from each side of the vagina and anastomose on the median line on the same path as the azygos arteries. The blood flow is oriented to uterine veins at the level of the cervix.

Veins are mainly located on the sides of the vagina and anastomose each other at the extremities of the vaginal canal. In the middle region of the vagina, anastomoses are carried out in the azygous arteries draining the blood to the uterine veins at the level of the cervix. The uterine veins are anastomosis with the average hemorrhoidal veins, which, in turn, communicate with the upper hemorrhoids, forming at this level a porta-cave anastomose. The *long vaginal vein* is the artery satellite of the same name when it exists, and it flows into the hypogastric vein.

6. Local hemodynamic changes during vaginal hysterectomy

- Vaginal hysterectomy has as its first step the disconnection of the upper vagina from the cervix and uterine body. As a result, the anastomotic flow between the uterus and vagina is interrupted.
- After the middle pedicles are cut, due to caudal traction of the cervix in the vaginal canal, the transversal segment of the uterine artery elongates, and it can be secured by occluding both the ascending and descending branch. After that, all the maneuverers in the uterus, until the upper pedicles, are bloodless.
- If the diameter of the uterus exceeds the lower pelvic brim, as the uterus is released, the bleeding is stopped by compressing the vessels on the hard plane of the pelvis.
- After extracting a large uterus, important bleeding may occur, caused by either ligature sliding or from the tearing of veins in the broad ligament.
- Many vaginal hysterectomies may result in insignificant bleeding as compared to those in abdominal hysterectomies.

Unlike abdominal hysterectomy, regardless of the method, open or laparoscopic, vaginal hysterectomy produces a particularly favorable effect by reducing bleeding, especially in the case of large uteri due to special hemodynamic conditions. During a vaginal hysterectomy, a series of hemodynamic events occur concerning the uterine circulation, especially for a large uterus:

Traction exerts on the cervix of a large uterus almost throughout the operation, so that blood flow is significantly diminished. After the bilateral ligature of the uterine arteries, which can affect both the ascending and the descending branches, the blood flow is completely stopped, allowing maneuvers for dimensional reduction of the uterus with no risk of significant bleeding.

During the vaginal hysterectomy, after the ligature of uterine arteries, visible bleeding does not come from vascular pedicles but from blood stored in the myometer.

7. Basic technique for vaginal hysterectomy

In cases where labia minora are hypertrophic and hinder access to the vaginal introit, they are anchored laterally by suture or by using the Richter retractor. The surgical area is bounded by a set of fields isolating the anterior vulval-perineal region (**Figure 8**).

8. Infiltration of vaginal wall

The course of the future colpotomy is infiltrated submucosally with a vasoconstrictive solution. (1/200,000 epinephrine, 4 ml of ropivacaine, and up to 20 ml of saline solution). When there are contraindications for administering the epinephrine, saline solution alone may be used. Through infiltration with saline solution, a hydric dissection of the tissues is achieved, which determines the opening of the cleavage spaces, and the local anesthesia blocks the nervous transmission from the receptor level.

Accidental intravascular injection should be avoided.

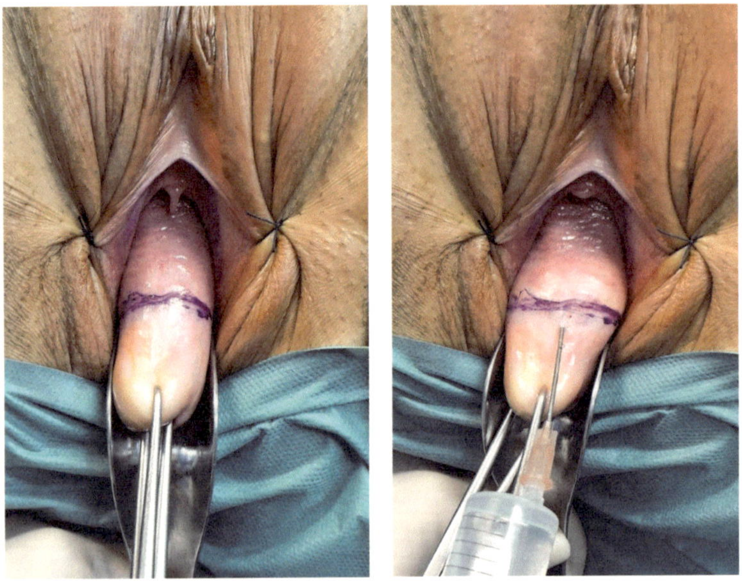

Figure 8.
Pericervical infiltration with saline solution. The cervix is grasped with 2 Pozzi clamps, and a magenta dye marks the limit of the anterior and posterior incision. Infiltrating is strictly submucosal.

8.1 Incision of the vagina around the cervix

The incision of the vaginal wall can be done with a cold or electric scalpel.

The incision of the vagina around the cervix is circular, with the anterior limit in the first transversal fold of the vaginal mucosa from its insertion into the cervix (*sulcus vesicalis*). The posterior limit should exceed the level of the cervical insertion of the two uterosacral ligaments (*torus uterinus*) in providing the closest access to open the pouch of Douglas. (see Chapter 6).

The incision includes the entire thickness of the vaginal wall, anteriorly and posteriorly. Laterally only the epithelium is interested. In this way, with the ligature of the first pedicle, the vagina will remain anchored sideways to the uterosacral ligaments, ensuring the prevention of the vaginal vault prolapse (**Figure 9**).

8.2 Developing anterior cleavage space (dissection of the bladder)

Entry into the anterior cleavage space starts with opening the vesicouterine space by cutting the *cervico-vesical septum.* After that, the vesicouterine space is entered digitally. In cases where there are scars after cesarean sections, it is recommended that the detachment be done with the scissors advancing less in the cervical plane or by "lateral window" (see Chapter 6) (**Figures 10** and **11**).

The peritoneal vesicouterine fold remains up as long as the uterus keeps its connections with the superior connective vascular pedicle. For this reason, its opening is not an immediate objective once the bladder has been detached from the uterus.

8.3 Opening the vesicouterine fold (anterior Colpoceliotomy)

In our basic technique, opening the vesicouterine pouch becomes extremely simple after the disconnection of the inferior pedicle if the uterus is not enlarged or deformed. After sectioning the inferior pedicle, the uterus descends 3–4 cm, where the white-pearly transversal fold of the peritoneal vesicouterine fold can be

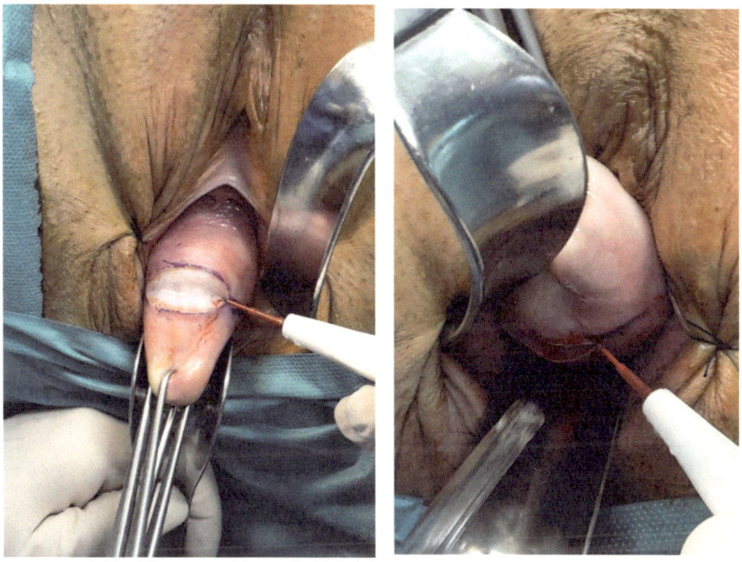

Figure 9.
The incision of the anterior wall of the vagina 1.5–2 cm away from the external cervical orifice includes the entire thickness of the vaginal wall. Posteriorly, the incision is placed at the level of the first posterior rugae of the vaginal wall.

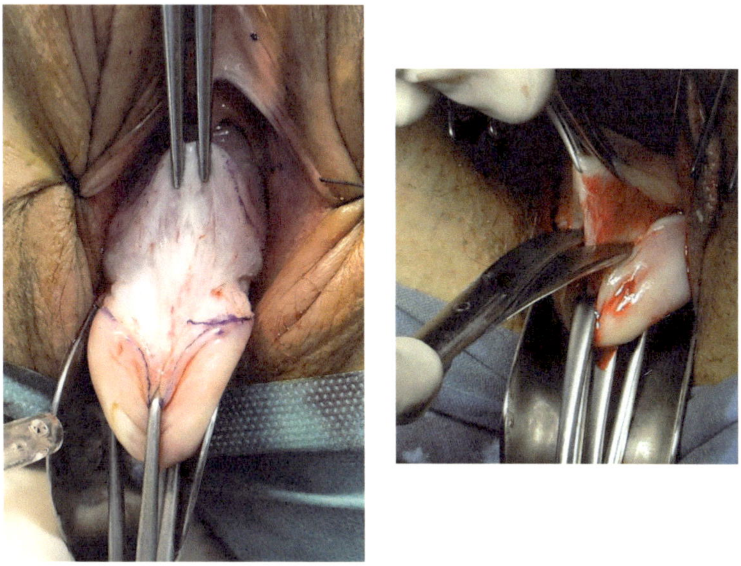

Figure 10.
To expose the cervico-vesical septum, the cervix is pulling down and the cutting edge of the vaginal wall in the opposite direction. The sectioning of the cervicovesical septum is done with scissors facing the mass of the cervix.

observed. It is grasped with a clamp and cut where it enters the pelvis. The surgeon digitally explores the anterior side of the uterus and inserts a Briesky-Navratil retractor in this space, discharging the bladder upward (**Figure 12**).

8.4 Developing rectovaginal space and opening the pouch of Douglas (posterior Colpoceliotomy)

Unlike with anterior colpoceliotomy, entering the rectovaginal cleavage space and opening the pouch of Douglas can be done at the same time. The level of

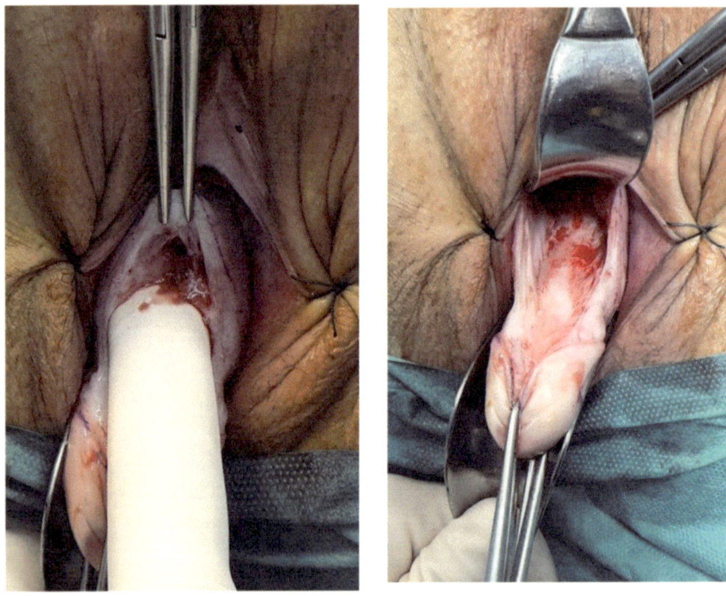

Figure 11.
The anterior cleavage space is open. Bladder pillars delineate the spatial side of anterior cleavage space. The dissection of the vesicouterine space is done by the progression of the index on the median line.

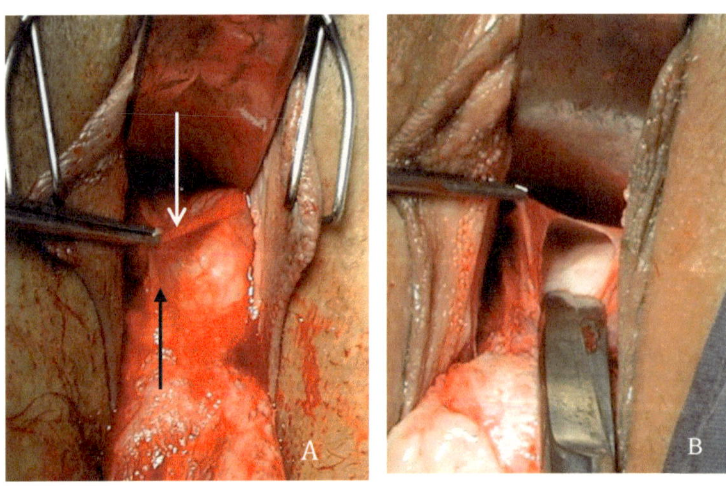

Figure 12.
A. Identifying and opening the real vesicovaginal fold (white arrow). The black arrow marks the cervical insertion of the peritoneal fold (false fold). B. the vesicovaginal fold opens.

posterior vaginal incision described above is significant to ensure a good entry into the rectovaginal space. The edge of the posterior vaginal wall incision is grasped with Allis clamps, and the rectovaginal space is entered by sharp or blunt dissection. After entering the rectovaginal space and pressing the rectum down, the peritoneal cul-de-sac may be observed swelling when the cervix is moved in or out. After opening the pouch of Douglas, the posterior side of the uterus, uterosacral ligaments, and the posterior leaf of the broad ligaments can be explored digitally (**Figures 13** and **14**).

In difficult cases, a particular variant can be used to avoid the creation of an excessively sizeable retroperitoneal space between the vagina and the rectum. (see Chapter 6).

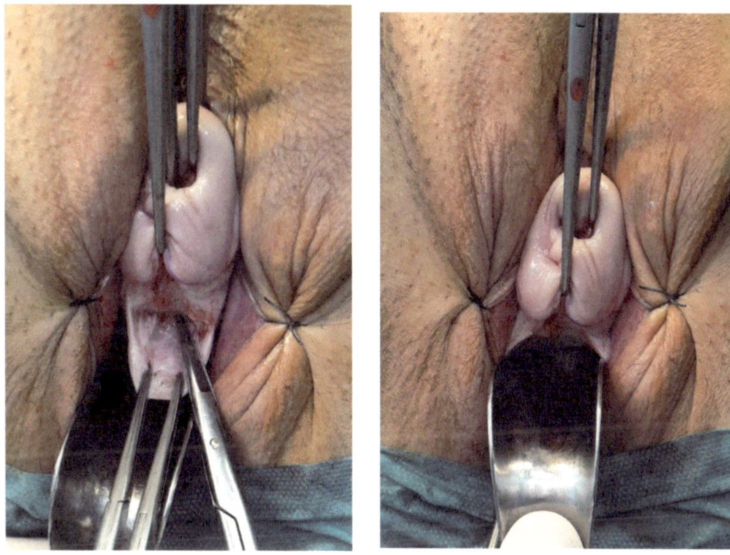

Figure 13.
Developing rectovaginal cleavage space. Allis clamps grasp the vaginal cutting edge, and the space is open by sharp dissection. The posterior aspect of the cervix is pulled upward, and the dissection is carried out using a Sims retractor.

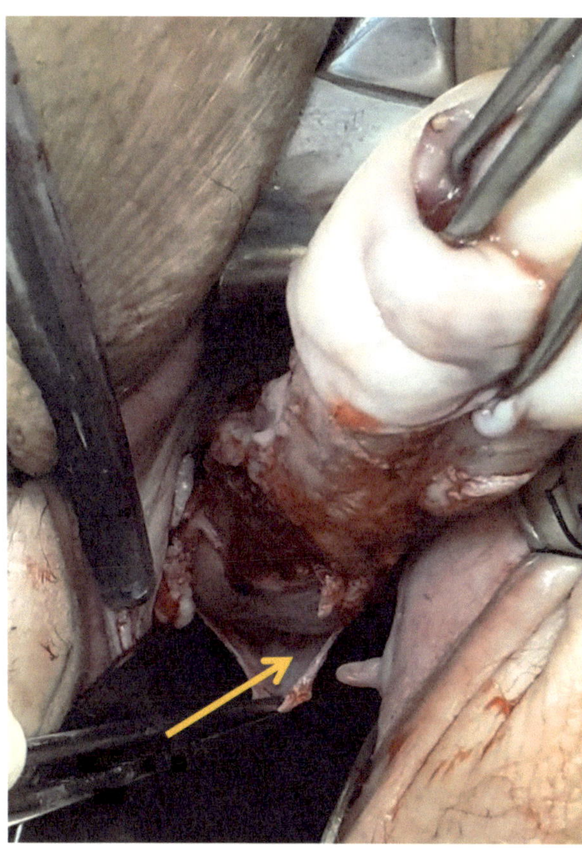

Figure 14.
The rectovaginal fold is open, and the posterior side of the uterus is visible. (arrow).

8.5 Disconnection of lower connective-vascular pedicle

The lower pedicle is represented by the uterosacral ligament posteriorly and the vesicouterine ligament anteriorly. For the disconnection of the inferior pedicle, it is not mandatory to open the rectouterine pouch, and the maneuver can be done extra-peritoneally.

The bladder is removed cranially with a Briesky-Navratil retractor, placing the two vesical pillars under tension, and the rectum is depressed with a posterior Sims retractor (**Figures 15** and **16**).

Using a Wertheim clamp, one of the uterosacral ligaments and the homologous bladder pillar are loaded together, after which, the pedicle is cut and ligated. The maneuver is repeated on the opposite side. In many situations, after cutting the pedicle, the pouch of Douglas opens spontaneously near the uterine edge.

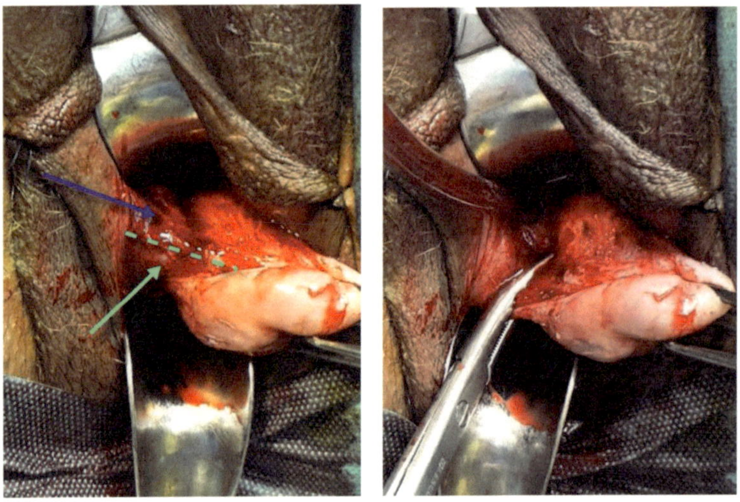

Figure 15.
Right lower pedicle. A dotted line separates the bladder pillar (blue arrow) from the uterosacral ligament (blue light arrow). Clamping the inferior part of the bladder pillar and uterosacral ligament together form the right lower pedicle.

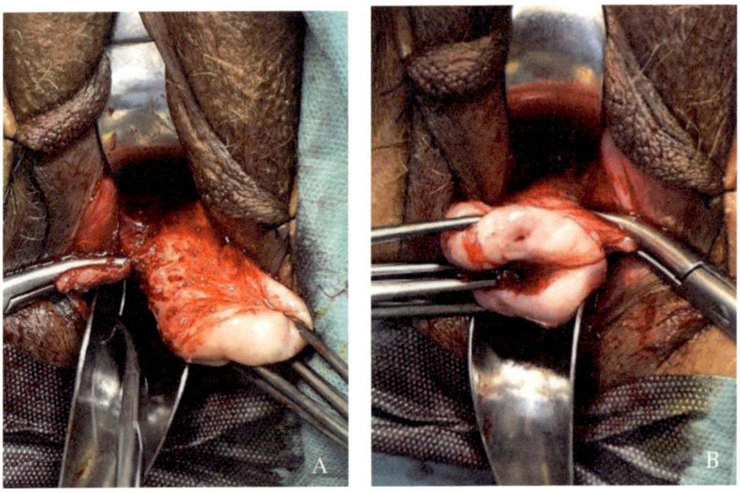

Figure 16.
A. Right lower pedicle secured by Vicryl 2/0. B. the left lower pedicle is clamped prepared to cut.

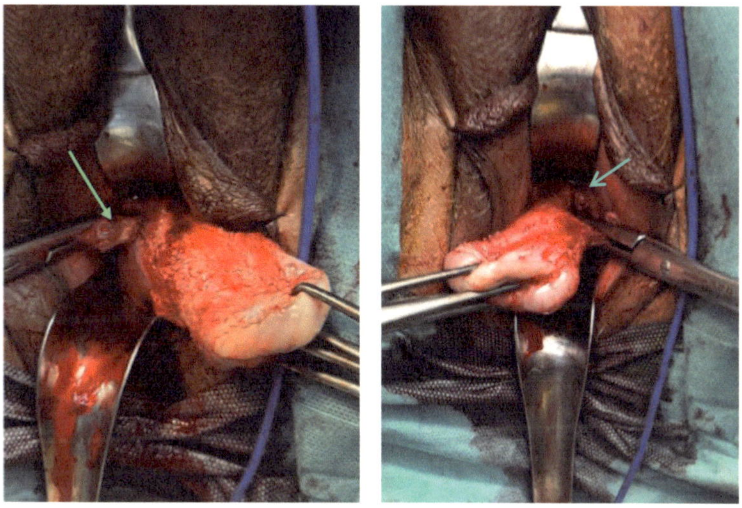

Figure 17.
Right middle pedicle formed by cardinal ligament and uterine artery and veins clamped and cut. Left middle pedicle clamped. Arrow mark the uterine artery. In our technique, the pediculisation of uterine vessels is not useful as long as the clamping of the pedicle is done strictly parallel to the uterine side. The risk to the ureter's damage is reduced if the lower pedicle is previously sectioned. (see chapter 2).

8.6 Disconnection of middle connective-vascular pedicle

The middle pedicle is represented by the cardinal ligament that contains the main uterine vascular supply for the uterus and cervix. By caudal traction on the cervix, the vascular pedicle has a parallel direction on the uterine edge, removing the ureters from the surgical field (**Figure 17**).

For this reason, during the vaginal hysterectomy, the urethral risk is lower than with the abdominal approach. After clamping, the pedicle is cut and ligated with 2–0 Vicryl.

In some situations, the cardinal ligament can be well represented and cannot be clamped at a single time. In this case, a second clamping and cutting should be cautiously be done. There is the risk of clamping and cutting a part of the superior pedicle and, in the maneuver, tilting the uterus. If so, the latter might break, causing some unwanted bleeding.

9. Disconnection of superior connective-vascular pedicle

For vaginally delivering the uterus, securing the superior connective vascular pedicle is the most important and sometimes the most difficult step of vaginal hysterectomy.

In most cases, the superior pedicle can be brought into the surgical field by tilting the uterus. The uterus can be tilted anteriorly (Doderlain-Kronig maneuver) or posteriorly (Heaney maneuver).

When the uterus is highly mobile and small, its release from the pelvis can also be done without tilting.

For the uterus weighing up to 200–280 g, access to the superior pedicle is done by tilting, a maneuver that brings the superior pedicle into the surgical field, which consists in anatomical order of the round ligament, fallopian tube, and homologous utero-ovarian ligament. This pedicle includes the anastomotic branch of the uterine artery and the tubo-ovarian vascular arch.

The main disadvantage of the tilting maneuvers is that it forces the vaginal opening through which the uterus is pulled, which can lead to the slipping of ligatures placed on the anteriorly cut and ligated connective vascular pedicles (**Figures 18–20**).

9.1 *Anterior tilting* (Doderlain-Kronig maneuver)

Anterior tilting (Doderlain-Kronig maneuver) is recommended in the case of a small uterus with a short superior pedicle or for a prolapsed uterus. The most common examples are those selected for vaginal subtotal hysterectomy. Anterior tilting is the quickest route to access the pedicle, but it cannot be used successfully with a large uterus (**Figure 21**).

The cervix is forcefully pulled caudally to expose as much as possible the anterior side of the uterus. Using a Pozzi clamp, the mass of the uterine body is clamped on the median line as high up as possible. It is gradually pulled, without sudden moves that lead to the rupture of the myometrium. At the same time, the cervix is left free without traction or pushed cranially and posteriorly with the Pozzi clamp. Along with the uterus's progress into the surgical field, using another Pozzi clamp, the mass of the uterine tissue is escalated as high up as possible until the uterine fundus and one or two superior pedicles appear in the surgical field. At this time, the cervix is pulled cranially to place the pedicle under tension. The index finger of the surgeon's left hand cranially and caudally loads the superior uterine pedicle, while the right-hand loads the pedicle into the arms of the Wertheim clamp.

After clamping and cutting, the pedicle is ligated, and the ends of the threads are kept as benchmarks. For the contralateral side, the maneuver for clamping the pedicle simplifies because, by pulling onto the cervix, the pedicle will be well exposed. Cutting and ligating the pedicles gives rise to the extraction of the uterus.

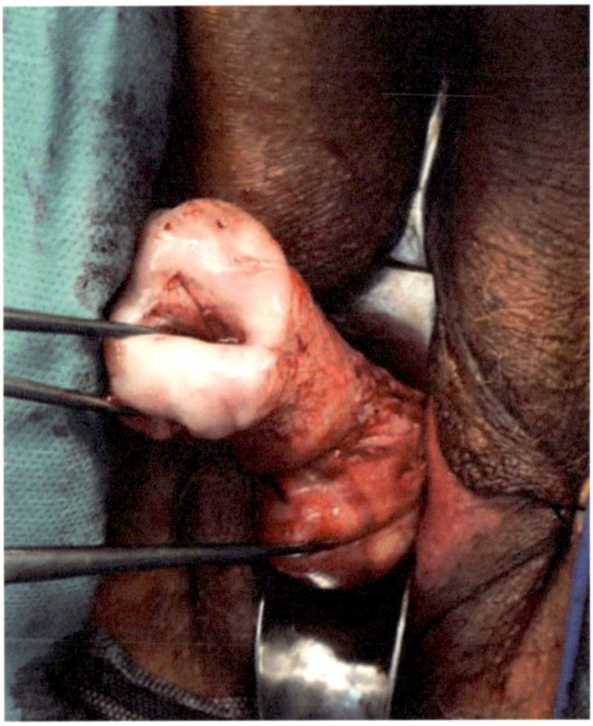

Figure 18.
Disconnection of upper pedicle by posterior tilting (Heaney maneuver).

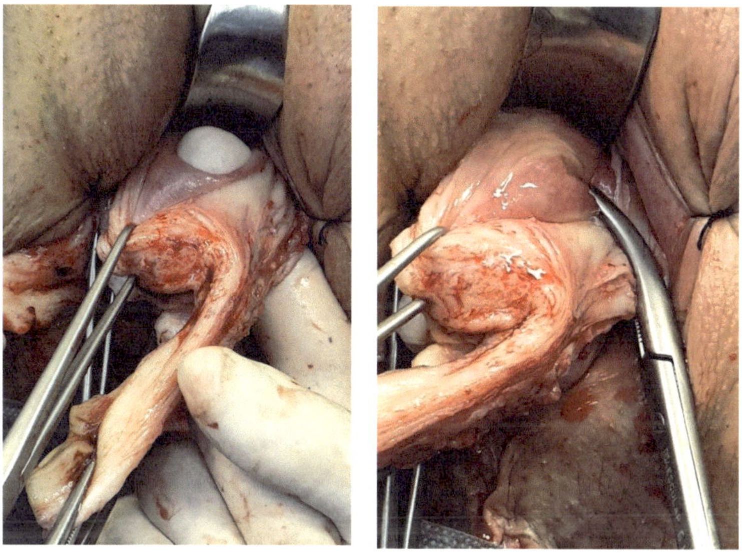

Figure 19.
Disconnection of the superior pedicle. In this case, the uterus is hemisected previously. The pedicle is hooked by the index finger and then clamped.

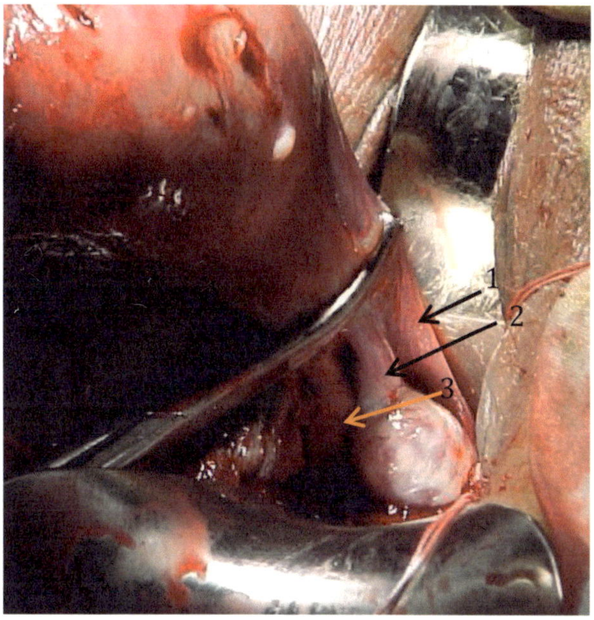

Figure 20.
Clamped left upper pedicle. We can see what it is made of 1 = round ligament, 2 = utero-ovarian ligament, 3 = tube.

The pedicle can be completely clamped or the round ligament isolated when one aims to perform the adnexectomy.

9.2 Posterior tilting (Heaney maneuver)

Posterior tilting (Heaney maneuver) is the most frequently used maneuver to access the superior pedicle for non-prolapsed uteruses weighing more than 180 g.

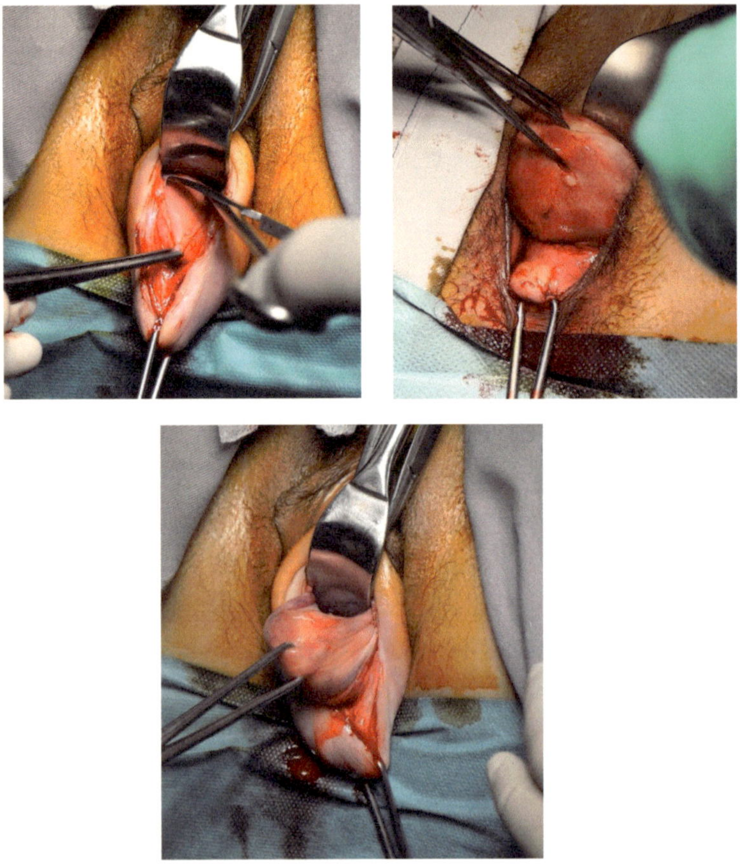

Figure 21.
Anterior tilting (Doderlain-Kronig maneuver). After anterior colpoceliotomy, the anterior side of the uterus is evident. Using Pozzi forceps, the uterine fundus is extracted, and the superior pedicle can be clamped and cut.

Posterior tilting has the main advantage of being able to rotate the uterus in a much larger space, represented by the sacral concavity.

The cervix is forcefully pulled cranially while the assistant depresses the rectum using a Sims retractor to reveal as much as possible of the posterior side of the uterus. The surgeon places a Pozzi clamp on the dorsal middle bottom of the uterus, as close as possible to the uterine pouch. Relaxing the tension exerted on the cervix, it is pulled progressively by the clamp while the assistant tries to extract the uterus using the posterior retractor. When uterus progression is observed, the position of the uterus pulling clamp is changed to become as cranial as possible, and the releasing maneuvers are continued until the uterine fundus appears in the surgical field (**Figures 22** and **23**).

Unlike anterior tilting, the superior pedicle does not become visible. To be able to identify it, the surgeon places a Briesky retractor in the area between the lateral wall of the vagina and the uterine horn, usually on the left side, where access is more accessible. As an aiding maneuver, the clamp anchoring the uterine fundus is repositioned as close as possible to the externalized uterine horn. Thus, by simultaneously pulling the cervix and uterine fundus and maneuvering the Briesky-Navratil retractor laterally, the superior pedicle is revealed at its insertion into the uterus. With the medius of the left hand, the surgeon loads the pedicle in a cranial position to clamp the pedicle in a caudal place with the right hand using a Wertheim clamp.

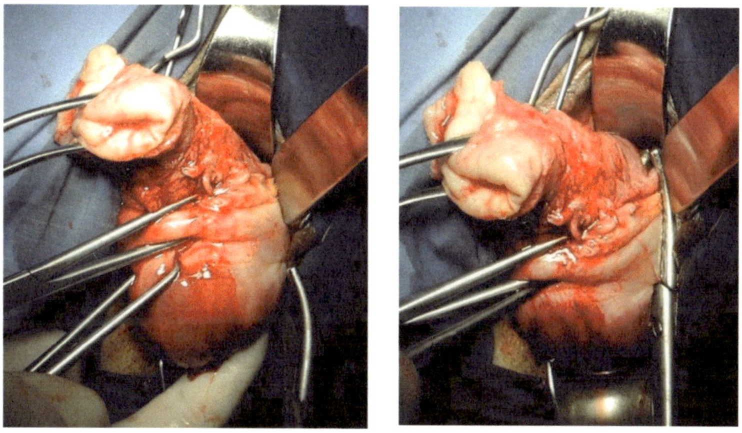

Figure 22.
Posterior tilting (Heaney maneuver). Clamping the left superior pedicle. The cervix is pulled cranially at the same time that the uterine fundus is pulled hard caudally.

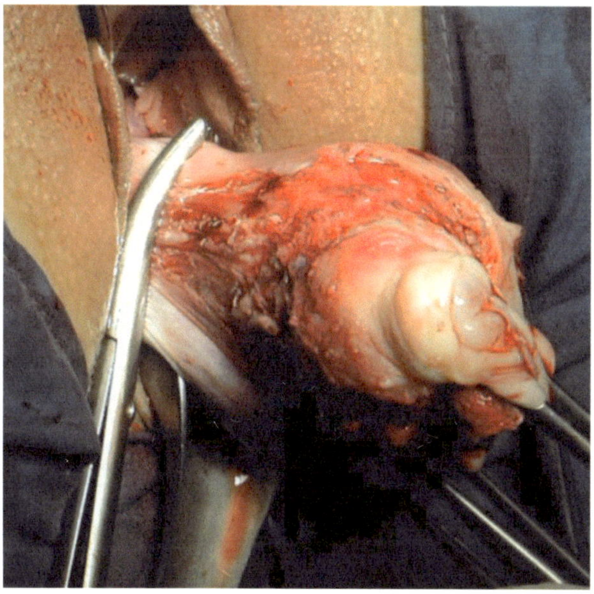

Figure 23.
The Heaney maneuver. The right pedicle is clamped "a la Vue easily. ".

9.3 Uterus release without tilting

In certain situations (early endometrial cancer, interventions under local anesthesia), it is necessary to release the uterus with minimum trauma, without tilting or morcellation. Direct access to the superior pedicle is possible mainly in multiparous women with perineal relaxation and small uteruses with a weakly represented bearing system. In these cases, clamping and section of the pedicle are done without any difficulties. Clamping the superior pedicle can be done safely by successively escalating the elements included in the utero-adnexal pedicle.

9.4 Bleeding control

After extracting the uterus, gauze is inserted through the vaginal opening and into the pelvic cavity, pushing the bowels and leaving the pelvic-subperitoneal space open to view. The posterior wall of the vagina is retracted with an auto-static retractor. The vesicouterine peritoneum is revealed using a Briesky-Navratil retractor. The basis of the parameter is shown on the appropriate side, pulling the thread locating the superior pedicle. Bleeding at the end of the intervention is usually profuse, and its primary source is the vaginal cutting edges. In the case of active arterial bleeding from parameters, the surgical field is flooded, and the primary sources, such as the uterine arteries or the utero-ovarian arches, are to be found immediately.

At the end of a vaginal hysterectomy, the surgical field is rarely "dry" until the vaginal cuff is closed.

9.5 Treatment of vaginal cuff

In the technique we used for a vaginal hysterectomy for a non-prolapsed uterus, we adopted the Wertheim manner of closing the peritoneal cavity and the remaining vaginal edges. The main drawback of this maneuver is the closing of the surgical field without controlling the hemostasis until the end of the operation. We modified the technique, closing down the pelvic-peritoneal space and anchoring the superior vagina to the remaining cuffs of the inferior pedicle containing the most substantial elements of suspension – the uterosacral ligaments. With this procedure, the prevention of vaginal vault prolapse is done like the McCall procedure.

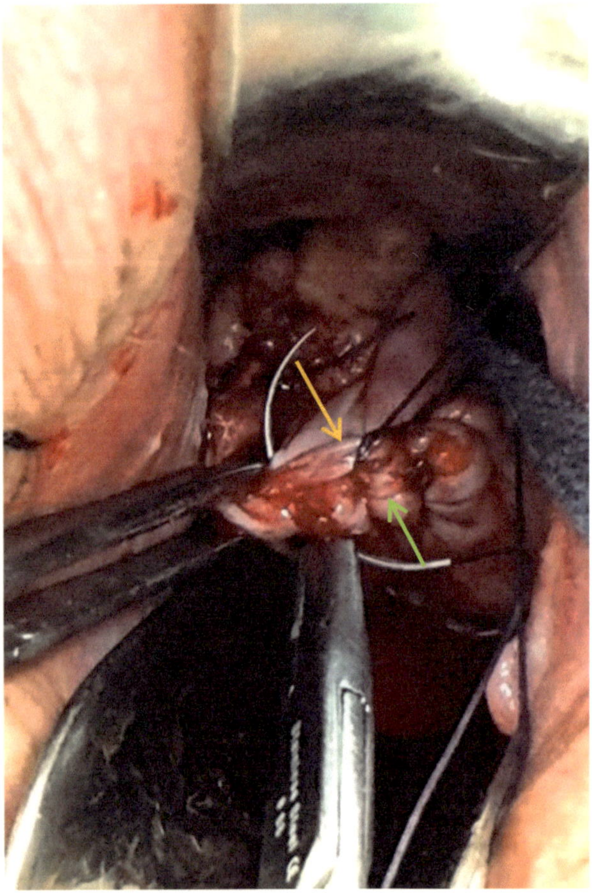

Figure 24.
Closing the posterior pelvic-subperitoneal space by running suture. The edge of the vagina (green arrow) is sutured together with the visceral posterior peritoneum (yellow arrow).

The manner we proposed is done in three distinct times:

- Closure of the pelvic-subperitoneal posterior space
- Closure of the pelvic-subperitoneal anterior space
- Full closure of the vaginal cuff

a. Closure of the pelvic-subperitoneal posterior space

Closing down the pelvic-subperitoneal space is done by running a suture with Vicryl nr. 0 to close the edge of the vagina and the posterior visceral peritoneum, starting from the lower pedicle on one side to the similar pedicle on the other side (**Figure 24**).

b. Closure of the pelvic-subperitoneal anterior space

This step usually is not necessary, but when the dissection of the bladder wall is difficult or in the case of an inadvertent wound, closing the space between the bladder and vagina is the best alternative. By joining the wall of the vagina with the visceral vesical peritoneum using a running suture, space is closed down.

c. Full closure of the vaginal cuff

The vaginal cuff can be fully closed by sutures with separate suture points. The closure of the vaginal cuff is done with Vicryl 0 and with

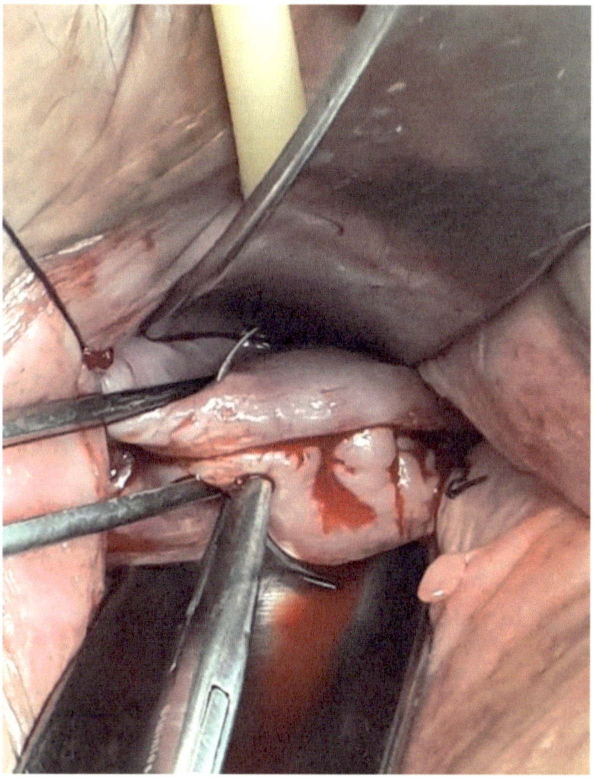

Figure 25.
The final closing of the vaginal vault by separate suture points, from middle to lateral.

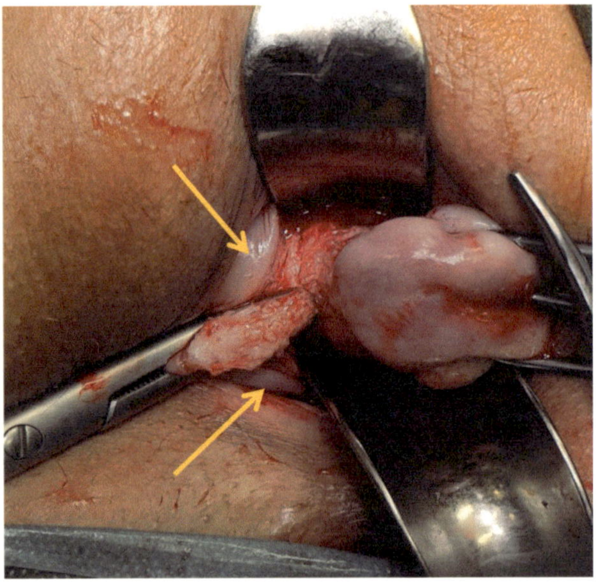

Figure 26.
Superficial incision of the lateral aspect of the vagina allows the section of the lower connective vascular pedicle to anchor the vaginal wall to uterosacral ligaments making prophylaxis of vaginal vault prolapse. (yellow arrows – Vaginal wall).

suture points in a figure of eight that starts at the center of the section and goes out towards each lateral vaginal commissure (**Figure 25**).

d. Prophylactic apical support

The technique described above refers to the unprolapsed uterus where post-hysterectomy vault prolapse occurs very rarely. For this reason, we do not include in the operative procedure an appropriate step addressed for it. The prevention of vaginal vault prolapse is necessary in case of an association of early forms of uterovaginal prolapse. By the technique described by us, the means of suspension of the upper vagina are preserved as long as the circular (**Figure 26**).

The incision in the cervix is of interest only to the vaginal mucosa. For cases where early apical prolapse is present, McCall culdoplasty is an excellent way to resuspend the upper vagina at the first level (DeLancey).

10. Conclusions at the end of the operation

The presented technique of vaginal hysterectomy resulted from combining several variants tried by authors over the years of more than 4500 vaginal hysterectomies. From each variant of the technique, we chose the most efficient and safe method to achieve each operator time as a confirmation of the validity of the succession of operating times proposed by us, the International Society of Endoscopic Surgery (ISGE) published in 2020 a set of recommendations on the technique of vaginal hysterectomy on the unprolapsed uterus.

Six recommendations were established similar to the standard technique proposed by us:

1. Circular incision at the level of the cervical-vagina junction is recommended (grade IC).

2. Posterior peritoneum should be opened first (grade IC).

3. Clamping and cutting the uterosacral and cardinal ligaments before or after getting access to the anterior peritoneum are recommended (grade IC).

4. Routine closure of the peritoneum during vaginal hysterectomy is not recommended (grade IB).

5. Vertical or horizontal closure of the vaginal vault following vaginal hysterectomy is recommended (grade IC).

6. To insert the vaginal plug following vaginal hysterectomy is not recommended (grade IB).

.., *Vaginal hysterectomy for a non-prolapsed uterus should be the preferred route for removing the uterus when hysterectomy is indicated. The ISGE provides evidence-based practical guidelines on how vaginal hysterectomy for non-prolapsed uterus should be undertaken. All efforts should be directed towards teaching the surgical technique of vaginal hysterectomy during residency.*

There is no standard technique for vaginal hysterectomies. Every case poses different strategical problems. It is not necessary to follow every step of the operation in order as described elsewhere in literature or even in this chapter. The surgeon can treat every operation as a distinct one with a specific strategy.

The disconnection of the leading vascular pedicles causes fewer problems than delivering the uterus from the upper connective vascular pedicle. For large uteri, this operative step is time-consuming and challenging to work for the surgeon.

If during the first steps of the operation, incidental bleeding begins that cannot be managed, the surgeon should not hesitate to convert the vaginal operation to an open abdominal or laparoscopic one. Every minute lost means 250 ml of blood lost from each uterine artery.

In many cases, there is significant blood loss until the uterus is released, and after that, the drama begins. In some cases, the abrupt withdrawal of the uterus from the pelvis causes the sliding of ligatures from a uterine artery. If the bleeding seems to be to one side, you have to look for it on the opposite side.

The most important thing is to finish this partially blind operation without any doubt regarding the safety of the patient.

Suggested reading

[1] Nichols DH, Randal CL. Vaginal Surgery. third ed. Williams &Wilkins; 1989

[2] Kovac SR, Zimmerman CV. Advances in Reconstructive Vaginal Surgery. Wolters Kluver, Lippincott, Williams & Wilkins; 2007

[3] Seth SS. Vaginal Hysterectomy. second ed. London: Jaypee Brothers Medical Publishers (P); 2014

[4] Cosson M, Querleu D, Dargent D. Vaginal Surgery. Taylor & Francis Group LLC; 2005

[5] Geller EJ. Vaginal hysterectomy: The original minimally invasive surgery. Minerva Ginecologica. 2014;**66**(1):23-33

[6] Bretschneider CE, Jallad K, Paraiso MFR. Minimally invasive hysterectomy for benign indications: An update. Minerva Ginecologica. 2017; **69**(3):295-303. DOI: 10.23736/S0026-4784.17.04017-5

[7] Chia KV, Tandon S, Moukarram H. Vaginal hysterectomy is made easier with ERBE Biclamp forceps. Journal of Obstetrics and Gynaecology. 2007; **27**(7):723-725. DOI: 10.1080/01443610701612789

[8] Purohit RK. Purohit technique of vaginal hysterectomy: A new approach. BJOG. 2003;**110**(12):1115-1119

[9] Rachaneni S, Dua A. Interventions to reduce morbidity from vault hematoma following vaginal hysterectomy: A systematic review and meta-analysis. International Urogynecology Journal. 2019;**30**(7):1061-1070. DOI: 10.1007/s00192-018-3829-6

[10] Von Theobald P, Grosdemouge I. Hystérectomie vaginale: technique opératoire caennaise Vaginal hysterectomy: operative technique used at Caen. Journal de Gynecologie, Obstetrique et Biologie de la Reproduction. 2002;**31**(6):589-596

[11] Chrysostomou A, Djokovic D, Edridge W, van Herendael BJ. Evidence-based practical guidelines of the International Society for Gynecologic Endoscopy (ISGE) for vaginal hysterectomy. European Journal of Obstetrics & Gynecology and Reproductive Biology. 2020;**252**

Author details

Petre Bratila
Minimally Invasive Gynecologic Excellence Center (SRC accreditated), Department of Robotic Surgery, Euroclinic Hospital, Bucharest, Romania

*Address all correspondence to: pbratila49@yahoo.com

Chapter 4

Laparoscopic Hysterectomy in Morbidly Obese Patients

Merima Ruhotina, Annemieke Wilcox, Shabnam Kashani and Masoud Azodi

Abstract

The following chapter will focus on laparoscopic hysterectomy in morbidly obese patients. The discussion reviews the physiological changes associated with morbid obesity and the potential implications on pneumoperitoneum during laparoscopic surgery. Important considerations such as perioperative care and operating room setup are discussed. Additionally, obtaining abdominal access, reviewing the surgical approach, and post-operative considerations are all highlighted within this chapter.

Keywords: minimally invasive surgery, morbid obesity, laparoscopic hysterectomy, robotic assisted laparoscopy hysterectomy

1. Introduction

Obesity worldwide has increased over time and is now considered an epidemic with significant health implications. Worldwide obesity has nearly tripled since 1975. In 2015–2016, the prevalence of obesity was 39.8% in adults and 18.5% in youth [1]. Body mass index (BMI) is a widely used method for estimating body fat mass. The World Health Organization defines class I obesity as BMI 30 to <35, class II obesity as BMI 35 to <40, and class III obesity as >40. The prevalence of clinically severe obesity (BMI > 40) is increasing at a much faster rate among adults in the United States than is the prevalence of moderate obesity [2]. In addition to the overall rising rates of severe obesity, the mean waist circumference (WC) has increased continuously among adults over the last 15 years. Abdominal fat deposition is a key component of obesity and some studies have shown that WC may be a better predictor for the risk of myocardial infarction, metabolic syndrome, and all-cause mortality than BMI [3].

From a surgical perspective, facilities need to consider the availability of specialized equipment for morbidly obese patients. Many facilities may lack the appropriate equipment for patient transfer, operating room tables that can accommodate the patient's weight, and specialized laparoscopic surgical equipment for minimally invasive surgery. Particular challenges of minimally invasive surgery for morbidly obese patients can be seen with central adiposity, which creates a thicker abdominal wall, larger visceral volume, and enlarged mesentaries, which can impact intraperitoneal visualization more difficult [4]. Central adiposity can also create technical challenges for entry into the abdominal cavity, difficulty with maneuvering laparoscopic instruments through a thick abdominal wall, and physiological stress of Trendelenburg position and pneumoperitoneum [5].

With respect to gynecologic minimally invasive surgery, obesity was previously considered a relative contra-indication. The first feasibility study of gynecologic laparoscopic surgery for obese patients was performed in 1976 [6]. With advances in minimally invasive technologies and increased operator experience, there has been growing evidence supporting minimally invasive surgery for obese patients. There is a large amount of data from gynecologic oncology indicating laparoscopic or robotic surgery resulted in shorter hospital stay, less postoperative pain, earlier return to normal activity, decreased postoperative complications, and fewer wound infections [7]. However, there are some studies indicating a higher conversion rate to laparotomy, which was dependent on BMI, noting that women who were morbidly obese had a 57% conversion rate to open laparotomy [8].

There is conflicting data regarding comparisons between robotic vs. conventional laparoscopic surgical outcomes. When looking at bariatric surgery studies, there is some evidence that robotic surgery results in shorter operative times with increased BMI [9]. However, other studies indicate that there are longer operative times [10]. One reason that surgeons may favor the use of robotic surgery is reduced surgeon fatigue, the utility of articulated wristed robotic instruments which allow for more fluid movements and less torque on the abdominal wall [11]. Further prospective studies are required to define the best and most cost-effective minimally invasive surgical method in obese women. Ultimately, every effort should be made to offer the least invasive procedure regardless of BMI, to maximize clinical benefits and quality of life [12].

2. Physiological changes

According to the National Institutes of Health, a BMI >40 increases the risk for diabetes mellitus, cardiovascular disease, and reduced life expectancy [13]. Understanding the differences in anatomy and physiology of morbidly obese patients is critical for surgical planning.

2.1 Cardiovascular

Myocardial infarction, cardiac failure, and sudden cardiac death risk increase in obese individuals. This may be due to increased body mass leading to hemodynamic and cardiovascular changes resulting in increased cardiac output, larger stroke volume, decreased vascular resistance, and increased cardiac workload [14]. In autopsy studies comparing obese and non-obese patients it has been found that obese patients can have 20–55% larger cardiac diameters, hypertrophied ventricles, and increased cardiac weight. These changes in cardiac physiology can result in hypertension and ultimately lead to cardiac failure [15]. Studies have found that ventricular hypertrophy and cardiac failure caused by obesity results in a higher risk of mortality [16]. The eccentric and concentric ventricular hypertrophy associated with obesity can lead to prolonged Q-T intervals or tachyarrhythmia. Additionally, unexplained cardiac arrhythmias are more common in obese patients [11]. The creation of pneumoperitoneum required to perform minimally invasive procedures can cause further cardiac depression. Abdominal insufflation causes an increase in afterload while the subsequent impeding of a venous return causes a decrease in preload. This contributes to an overall reduction in cardiac output [17]. Cardiac depression during laparoscopic procedures is often transient as the patient's body compensates for the change in physiology. In one study of morbidly obese patients undergoing laparoscopic gastric bypass, cardiac output levels returned to baseline at 2.5 hours after abdominal insufflation [17].

2.2 Pulmonary

Due to fat deposits in the mediastinum and abdominal cavities, the mechanical properties of the lungs and chest wall are altered in obese patients resulting in reduced compliance of the lungs, chest wall, and entire respiratory system. These changes likely contribute to increased symptoms of wheezing, dyspnea, and orthopnea [18]. Obesity causes reduced chest wall and pulmonary compliance and therefore reduction in gas exchange and increased bronchial resistance and ventilation-perfusion. Increased abdominal pressure and pleural pressures in obesity alter the breathing pattern resulting in a reduction of both expiratory reserve volume (ERV) and the functional residual capacity (FRC). Severely obese patients have a decreased FRC up to 33% [11, 18].

The expiratory reserve volume is also compromised by 35–60%, secondary to cephalad displacement of the diaphragm by the obese abdomen [19]. Sleep-disordered breathing, including obstructive sleep apnea (OSA) and obesity-related respiratory failure (ORRF) is common in obese patients. Studies demonstrated that half of all patients with a BMI >40 kg/m^2 demonstrate OSA [20]. Untreated OSA can result in hypoxemia during sleep as well as pulmonary hypertension, both of which increase risk of cardiac arrythmias. In addition, OSA has been associated with postoperative respiratory complications pneumonia, postoperative hypoxemia, and unplanned reintubation [11].

There are additional intrinsic qualities of an obese body habitus that can impair respiratory function. More soft tissue of the upper airway combined with increased tongue size can cause significant upper airway resistance [16]. An increase in breast mass and additional adiposity can cause difficulty with direct laryngoscopy [16]. Finally, a waist-to-hip ratio has been found to poorly impact gas exchange with larger waist-to-hip ratios correlating to worsening arterial blood gas values [11, 16, 21].

Performing a minimally invasive hysterectomy requires the patient to undergo general anesthesia, the creation of pneumoperitoneum, and supine positioning, all of which further impact respiratory physiology in obese patients. The administration of general anesthesia can reduce a patient's FRC by an additional 20%, while pneumoperitoneum increases inspiratory resistance requiring higher minute ventilation [11, 15]. In one study evaluating respiratory mechanics in laparoscopy, it was found that obese, anesthetized patients in the supine position required 15% higher minute ventilation to maintain normocarbia prior to abdominal insufflation. The authors also reported that these patients had 30% lower static compliance and 68% higher inspiratory resistance after insufflation of the abdomen with CO2 to a pressure of 20 mmHg [15, 22]. While the increase in inspiratory restitance caused by obesity requires higher minute ventilation, oxygenation does not seem to be affected by abdominal insufflation or Trendelenburg positioning. Therefore, patients who are able to tolerate general anesthesia in the supine position are likely also able to tolerate abdominal insufflation and changes in position including Trendelenburg [15, 22].

2.3 Gastrointestinal system

Gastric and esophageal function may also be impaired in obese patients, which can lead to intra-operative challenges. Gastroesophageal reflux disease (GERD) and hiatal hernias are found more commonly in obese patients and can often be asymptomatic [11]. This is caused by increased intra-abdominal pressure which can be two to three times higher in morbidly obese patients compared with non-obese patients [11]. Studies have found that obese patients tend to have higher gastric volumes, lower gastric pH, and delayed emptying which can increase their risk of intra-operative and post-operative gastric acid aspiration [11, 15]. For this reason, a prophylactic H2 blocker (ranitidine) and a pro-kinetic (metoclopramide) are often recommended prior to a surgical procedure [16].

2.4 Thromboembolism

Obesity is an independent risk factor for venous thromboembolism (VTE). Current data regarding the risk of VTE in gynecologic surgery shows the incidence of VTE in gyn surgery ranges from 0 to 2%. Evidence for these studies is from retrospective studies in non-obese patients who underwent simple laparoscopic procedures [11]. Gynecologic laparoscopic procedures with a duration of >30 min are considered moderate to high risk for VTE. Increasing laparscopic surgical complexity increases rates of VTE after completion of surgery according to the American College of Chest Physicians (ACCP) [23]. For these procedures, the standard treatment for VTE prophylaxis is mechanical prophylaxis with sequential compression devices. For obese patients it is critical these devices are appropriately fitted. Alternatively, pharmacologic prophylaxis with either subcutaneous low molecular weight heparin or unfractionated heparin can be administered. For bariatric surgery patients who have a BMI >55, immobility, history of active or recent VTE, hypercoagulable disorders, or severe OSA there are recommendations for placement of an inferior vena cava (IVC) filter for patients prior to bariatric surgery [24]. There are no current clear guidelines for patients undergoing gynecologic laparoscopic surgery and decisions should be made on an individual basis. The ACCP recommends dual prophylaxis with sequential compression devices and pharmacologic prophylaxis during admission and prolonged pharmacologic prophylaxis for 2–4 weeks after discharge for patients with gynecologic cancer with additional risk factors such as age >60 or history of VTE [23]. Recommendations for patients who are morbidly obese undergoing gynecologic laparoscopy may include combination mechanical and pharmacological prophylaxis during surgery and hospitalization. Taking into consideration patient comorbidities and mobility status, extended prophylaxis after discharge may also be considered [11].

3. Perioperative considerations

It is imperative that morbidly obese patients who are seen for surgical consultation should have a comprehensive history and physical exam in addition to laboratory and diagnostic testing as their obesity can increase their medical complexity. During a physical exam, there should be documentation of the patient's body habitus, assessment of the uterine size, uterine mobility, and vaginal caliber. Proper evaluation of the patient's panniculus and body type is crucial for determining intravenous access, trocar placement, and positioning during laparoscopy [4]. Special attention must be paid to the distribution of the patient's weight (i.e. increased waist circumference vs. increased hip circumference). Patients with large adipose tissue centered on their waist are likely to be more technically challenging than patients whose adipose is centered on the hips [15]. In patients with large panniculus, trocar placement may be hindered not only by increased thickness but also by a lack of mobility. If the panniculus is soft and mobile, it can be repositioned easily using traction with weights or tape.

In general, preoperative testing should be tailored to the patient's risk factors. Basic laboratory assessment can include a complete blood count, blood glucose concentration, basic metabolic panel, and blood type and screening. Given the high predisposition for cardiovascular, pulmonary, and endocrine abnormalities in morbidly obese patients, evaluation by subspecialists for additional diagnostic testing should be performed. Informed consent should take into account both the increased medical and surgical complexity of the case and inform the patient of increased risk of infection, increased risk of VTE, and potential increased risk for conversion to laparotomy [11]. As pulmonary and cardiovascular changes are prominent in morbidly obese patients, there are numerous risks associated with general anesthesia including airway complications and oxygenation issues with induction of anesthesia, intubation, and extubation [4]. Increased communication with anesthesia and pre-operative evaluation with anesthesia may be beneficial for these patients. When considering antibiotic prophylaxis, the current standard for routine prophylaxis prior to hysterectomy is 2 g of cefazolin for patients under 120 kg and 3 g for patients over 120 kg [25]. With regards to mechanical bowel prep (MBP), the theoretical advantage is to reduce intestinal volume and mass to improve intraoperative manipulation and visualization. A meta-analysis of elective colorectal surgery has revealed no statistical advantage of MBP [4].

4. Operating room setup

In order to complete laparoscopic surgery safely and efficiently for morbidly obese patients, proper preparation in the operating room is essential. Proper setup of the operating room will allow for mobility of the surgical team, quick access to instruments, increase patient safety, and the ability for the surgeon to successfully complete the procedure.

The first consideration needs to be placed on basic operating room equipment such as the operating room table and mechanisms for patient transfer. Patients are usually brought to the operating room in a stretcher. Lateral transfer devices that utilize hover technology (Hovermatt) can enable the team to move the patient to the operating room table and back to the transport stretcher in a secure and comfortable manner [26]. Operating room tables must have the capacity to support morbidly obese patients. Many standard tables have weight limits of 227 kg (500 lb). A bariatric bed is wider than traditional beds and can accommodate a weight of up to 1000 lb. If there is no availability of a bariatric bed, two standard operating room tables can be used together. Extra padding, blankets, sheets, or lifting devices may be needed to appropriately position an obese patient. Blood pressure cuffs and sequential compression devices will need to be of appropriate size to provide accurate readings.

An additional consideration should be placed on specialized laparoscopic instruments. Laparoscopes come in various sizes with a standard length of 32 cm and diameters ranging from 2 to 10 mm. There are various angled scopes available. In bariatric surgery, some surgeons endorse using a 45-degree angled scope or an extra-long laparoscope (45 cm) to aid with viewing flexibility in extremely obese patients [27]. Laparoscopic assist trays may include extra-long laparoscopic instruments (41–45 cm), which may aid with the ability to complete the procedure successfully. Instruments such as long trocars, trocars with a non-latex balloon at the distal end for retention of the trocar tip in the abdominal cavity, or a long Veress needle (150 mm) may be used. Uterine manipulators should be considered for safe completion of hysterectomy. Although redundant perineal tissue or a large uterus may limit the full mobility of the uterus, the integrated cervical cup will allow for cephalad traction and proper identification of surgical landmarks for colpotomy creation and increase the distance of the uterine arteries from the ureters [4].

5. Patient positioning

Obese patients are at greater risk for pressure sores and nerve injuries when compared to non-obese patients. Duration of compression and compressive force applied influence the risk of nerve injuries. Prolonged compression for 6–8 hours can cause permanent nerve injuries [11, 28, 29]. For laparoscopic surgical procedures in gynecology, patients are placed in a dorsal lithotomy position with their arms tucked at their sides in a "military" position. It is recommended to initially position the buttocks slightly lower than the edge of the bed as the body will shift cephalad with the weight of the panniculus once in Trendelenburg position.

Several considerations should be taken when tucking the arms. It is important to ensure that all intravenous access and cardiopulmonary monitors are functioning appropriately. Adequate padding should be placed at the hands and elbows to minimze ulnar or branchial plexus injuries [29]. If the arms are hanging too far off the side of the bed, bed extenders or arm sleds can be used. If the patient slides cephalad with shoulder blocks in place or if the arms are extended. Two potential scenarios that can increase the risk of brachial plexus injury are if the patient slides cephalad with shoulder blocks in place or if the surgeon leans on the patient's extended arms [30]. The legs should be positioned in stirrups in a low lithotomy position with generous padding applied around the hips and knees. The most common stirrups available in the United States are the YellowFin, the YelloFin Elite, and the Ultrafin. The Ultrafin is capable of accommodating calves that are 13 inches wide and have a weight capacity of 800 lb. Appropriate selection of stirrups can potentially aid in decreasing nerve injury. Obese patients have an increased risk for brachial plexus injury given downward shifting in Trendelenburg [11]. There are multiple options to help reduce this cephalad shifting including gel padding, egg-crate foam, surgical bag, and a padded straps. Once the patient has been positioned a "tilt-test" can be performed where the patient is placed into Trendelenburg position for approximately 2–5 minutes in order to assess the stability of the patient's positioning and assess the impact on the respiratory and cardiac status. Some adjustments that can be made to help insufflation pressures would be to decrease the degree of Trendelenburg or reduce the insuflation pressure.

6. Panniculus management

Management of the patient's panniculus in a caudad position during laparoscopic surgery can aid in improving the patient's ventilation and therefore potentially decreasing the conversation to laparotomy. One technique involves the use of a foley catheter that is passed through the patient's abdominal wall. The foley balloon is insuflated and the catheter is pulled up and clamped to a retractor attached to the foot of the bed [31]. A second technique involves using towel clips on the lower edge of the panniculus with 1-liter saline bags attached and hanging between the legs. Lastly, adhesive dressing can be used to secure the panniculus to the patient's thighs.

7. Abdominal access

Morbid obesity can increase the difficulty of initial abdominal access in laparoscopic surgery due to the increased thickness of the abdominal wall and lack of reliable landmarks. Traditionally, the umbilicus is a common landmark used for abdominal entry as it may represent the thinnest part of the abdominal wall.

However, in obese patients, the umbilicus is often located at or cephalad to the aortic bifurcation. In obese women, the mean umbilical location was found to be on average 2.9 cm caudal to the aortic bifurcation in comparison to nonobese women in which the umbilicus was 0.4 cm caudual to the bifurcation [32]. Given this migration of the umbilicus, if it is used for entry into the abdomen, it may compromise adequate triangulation with the surgical pathology [11]. There are multiple techniques for abdominal entry including the Veress needle, use of an optical trocar, or an open technique. In obese patients, there is a higher likelihood for the Veress technique to result in a higher rate of false entry and preperitoneal insufflation [11]. If there is no substantial panniculus and the umbilical approach is chosen, a 90-degree entry can be used and the use of a long Veress needle (150 mm) may help decrease pre-peritoneal insufflation. If an optical trocar is used, it may be beneficial to use a long trocar to aid in correct placement. Supraumbilical and left upper quadrant are two alternative abdominal entry sites. If the left upper quadrant is used, a nasogastric or orogastric drainage tube should be placed to decompress the stomach. This site is contraindicated in patients who have a history of gastric bypass, splenectomy, and splenomegaly.

8. Surgical approach

Obesity is an important factor to consider when determining an appropriate surgical approach to hysterectomy. A systematic review published in 2015 by Blikkendaal et al., found that laparoscopic hysterectomy and vaginal hysterectomy are associated with significantly fewer postoperative complications and shorter lengths of hospital stay [31]. While vaginal hysterectomy is generally the preferred surgical approach and is associated with improved outcomes, it seems to be less favorable in obese patients due to large uterine size, early-stage endometrial cancer, or lack of vaginal access and exposure secondary to the patient's body habitus [31]. In patients who are not good candidates for vaginal surgery, conventional laparoscopic hysterectomy and robotic hysterectomy are alternative approaches that are shown to be safe and feasible in this patient population [31, 32].

The benefits of minimally invasive surgery are well studied. Compared to laparotomy, laparoscopic hysterectomy results in fewer postoperative complications, decreased blood loss, less time in the hospital, and faster recovery [31, 33]. One study showed that obese patients who underwent laparoscopic hysterectomy compared with laparotomy had fewer incidences of postoperative ileus (0% vs. 13.3%), less postoperative fevers (5.5% vs. 31.1%), and a decrease in wound infections (9% vs. 22%) [15]. Additionally, obese women undergoing laparoscopic hysterectomies, bilateral salpingo-oophorectomy, and lymph node dissection for stage I endometrial carcinoma were found to have shorter hospital stays (2.5 vs. 5.6 days), less pain (32.2 vs. 124.1 mg of pain medication), and earlier return to normal activity [15].

Despite the clear benefits of minimally invasive techniques, research evaluating surgeons' surgical preference shows that the rate of abdominal hysterectomy increases as BMI increases [31]. In fact, in the past obesity was considered a relative contraindication to laparoscopic surgery. This is due to associated difficulties with Verees needle placement, accumulation of fat in the omentum obstructing the operative field and manipulation of laparoscopic instruments [15]. However, more recent studies have shown that minimally invasive approaches including robotics and conventional laparoscopic techniques can be successful in obese patients with proper planning and appropriate laparoscopic surgical experience.

Robotic surgery may help overcome some of the inherent challenges of minimally invasive surgery in obese patients. Robotic surgery offers greater flexibility, articulation, and control of the instruments with reduced hand tremors. Improved ergonomics and the 3D-HD view allow for surgeons to more easily operate within the confined space of an obese abdomen and reduce surgeon fatigue [33]. This is especially relevant in obese patients with endometrial cancer when lymphadenectomy is required [34]. The advantages of robotic surgery may help facilitate the completion of hysterectomy using a minimally invasive approach, however, the cost is significant. Each robotic console has a direct cost of $2.6 million USD and about $2000 per surgical case [34].

While most studies comparing robotic surgery to laparoscopic surgery have not been able to show an improvement in safety or efficacy compared with conventional laparoscopy, there is evidence that robotic surgery may provide clinical benefits in specific populations like the morbidly obese [34–36]. In fact, there is evidence of cost neutralization with robotic procedures when the rate of conversion to laparotomy is decreased [34]. A recent systematic review and meta-analysis comparing laparoscopic and robotic hysterectomy in endometrial cancer patients with obesity found similar perioperative complication rates but a decrease in conversion to laparotomy in robotic procedures performed on patients with BMI > 40 kg/m^2 (7.0% vs. 3.8%) [34]. Additionally, the qualitative reasons for conversion were different in robotic hysterectomy and conventional laparoscopic hysterectomy. Conversion to laparotomy from conventional laparoscopy was more often due to obesity-related anesthetic concerns (30% vs. 6%) while conversion from robotic assisted laparoscopy was attributed more frequently to increased uterine size [34].

9. Intraoperative considerations

9.1 Trocar placement

After properly positioning the patient and obtaining adequate pneumoperitoneum, the surgeon must determine adequate and safe port site placement. This step can be more challenging in obese patient as traditional landmarks may be altered. The surgeon should choose trocars that are adequate in length. Although extra-long trocars, up to 150 mm, are available and may be useful in patients with very thick anterior abdominal walls, they are often not necessary [29, 37]. In order to safely place accessory trocars, some authors recommend increasing the insufflation pressure to 25 mmHg to increase the distance for trocar placement in order to avoid vascular and visceral complications [37]. Once the initial trocar is placed and pneumoperitoneum is achieved, ancillary trocars can be placed under direct visualization after localization with a spinal needle [37]. In general, most authors recommend more cephalad and lateral placement of ancillary port in obese women. This is due to the difficult visualization of the inferior epigastric vessels and the extent of the panniculus [11, 29, 38]. When placing ancillary trocars, they should be angled toward the operative field to prevent slippage and torquing of the instruments [15]. Surgeons should have a low threshold for adding additional ports that may improve ergonomics, triangulation, or retraction [29, 38].

9.2 Exposure and uterine manipulation

Surgical exposure can be challenging in obese patients. This is due to increased visceral adiposity, a fatty rectosigmoid colon, or limited Trendelenburg positioning due to difficulty with ventilation [29, 32]. Mobilizing the cecum and sigmoid reflection from their lateral peritoneal attachments can help facilitate moving the large bowel out of the pelvis [29]. Additionally, the rectosigmoid colon can be retracted by using a puppet stitch to pull the epiploic appendices to the anterior abdominal wall [11]. Another option is using a pre-tied endoscopic loop that can be brought through the anterior abdominal wall using a fascial closure device or bringing the suture through a trocar to be tied off [29, 38].

Effective uterine manipulation is especially important to perform laparoscopic and robotic hysterectomies safely in obese patients. This is because the amount of Trendelenburg may be limited and exposure to the pelvis may be challenging [37]. There are many uterine manipulation devices available including the Zinnati Uterine Manipulator injector (ZUMI) (Cooper Surgical, Trumball, CT), the VCare (ConMed Endosurgery, Utica, NY), and the Reusable Uterine Manipulator Injector (RUMI) Arch (Cooper Surgical, Trumball, CT). It is recommended that surgeons choose a device that will be applicable to the majority of their cases so that the entire surgical team can become familiar with its use, allowing for reliable uterine manipulation [37].

9.3 Closure techniques

As with non-obese patients, closure of the fascia is recommended in incisions greater than 10 mm to prevent port site evisceration. Exposure to the fascia can be more challenging in obese patients. Facial closure devices like the reusable Carter-Thomason CloseSure System XL device (Cooper Surgical, Trumball, CT) allow for the closure to be performed under direct visualization. If the device is not long enough, the disposable Endoclose device (Covidien, Norwalk, CT) can be used [37].

Many studies have compared vaginal vs. laparoscopic vaginal cuff closure with more recent data showing a reduction in vaginal cuff dehiscence with laparoscopic closure (1% vs. 2.7%) [24]. A study by Uccella et al. further demonstrated a reduction in vaginal bleeding (2.7% vs. 4.9%), vaginal cuff hematoma (0.9% vs. 2.3%), need for vaginal re-suturing (0.9% vs. 2.3%) and postoperative infection (0.9% vs. 2.3%) [39]. In obese patients with limited vaginal access due to weight distribution or a large panniculus, laparoscopic closure may also be more accessible.

Some research suggests that obesity may be a protective factor against vaginal cuff dehiscence and evisceration. One study found that after laparoscopic hysterectomy, obese women were 86% less likely to experience vaginal cuff dehiscence than non-obese women [40, 41]. Although intercourse is a significant risk factor for cuff dehiscence, it is hypothesized that positioning during intercourse may be different for obese women, resulting in the application of less physical force at the apex of the vagina [40, 41]. The authors further also postulate that an increase in adipose tissue leads to less energy being delivered to the vaginal tissue during the creation of colpotomy, which can improve healing by causing less tissue desiccation.

10. Post-operative care

Studies have shown that the incidence of postoperative complications increases as BMI increases. However, when surgeries are performed in a minimally invasive fashion, complication rates for obese patients are similar to non-obese patients [29].

Patients with known or presumed cardiovascular disease, OSA, or high perioperative risk should be monitored closely in the postoperative period. Patients who have OSA should be observed overnight because of the increased risk of pulmonary complications [11, 29]. A multi-modal approach to analgesia is recommended to limit narcotic analgesic which can worsen atelectasis and hypoxia. This may include acetaminophen, nonsteroidal anti-inflammatory agents, cyclooxygenase-2 inhibitors, gabapentin, or pregabalin as well as local or regional anesthesia [29, 42]. Early ambulation and the use of incentive spirometry can help inflate dependent lung regions and decrease impairment of lung function induced by anesthesia. As discussed above in the thromboembolism section of this chapter, morbidly obese patients are at increased risk for VTE and may benefit from from extended VTE prophylaxis for 10–35 days following surgery [11, 23].

11. Conclusion

Minimally invasive laparoscopic hysterectomy is feasible for morbidly obese patients. Additional considerations regarding cardiopulmonary physiological changes seen in morbid obesity should be stressed as these have implications for preoperative surgical risk assessment and the patient's ability to tolerate surgical positioning and pneumoperitoneum.

Author details

Merima Ruhotina*, Annemieke Wilcox, Shabnam Kashani and Masoud Azodi
Yale New Haven Health Bridgeport Hospital, Yale School of Medicine, United States

*Address all correspondence to: merima.ruhotina@yale.edu

References

[1] Hales CM, Carroll MD, Fryar CD, Ogden CL. Prevalence of obesity among adults and youth: United States, 2015-2016. NCHS Data Brief. 2017;**288**:1-8

[2] Sturm R. Increases in morbid obesity in the USA: 2000-2005. Public Health. 2007;**121**(7):492-496. DOI: 10.1016/j.puhe.2007.01.006. Epub 2007 Mar 30

[3] Li C, Ford ES, McGuire LC, Mokdad AH. Increasing trends in waist circumference and abdominal obesity among US adults. Obesity (Silver Spring). 2007;**15**(1):216-224. DOI: 10.1038/oby.2007.505

[4] Menderes G, Gysler SM, Vadivelu N, Silasi DA. Challenges of robotic gynecologic surgery in morbidly obese patients and how to optimize success. Current Pain and Headache Reports. 2019;**23**(7):51. DOI: 10.1007/s11916-019-0788-7

[5] Lee WJ, Wang W, Chen TC, Wei PL, Lin CM, Huang MT. Clinical significance of central obesity in laparoscopic bariatric surgery. Obesity Surgery. 2003;**13**(6):921-925. DOI: 10.1381/096089203322618786

[6] Loffer FD, Pent D. Laparoscopy in the obese patient. American Journal of Obstetrics and Gynecology. 1976; **125**(1):104-107. DOI: 10.1016/0002-9378(76)90902-9

[7] Eltabbakh GH, Piver MS, Hempling RE, Recio FO. Laparoscopic surgery in obese women. Obstetrics and Gynecology. 1999;**94**(5 Pt 1):704-708. DOI: 10.1016/s0029-7844(99)00406-8

[8] Walker JL, Piedmonte MR, Spirtos NM, Eisenkop SM, Schlaerth JB, Mannel RS, et al. Laparoscopy compared with laparotomy for comprehensive surgical staging of uterine cancer: Gynecologic Oncology Group Study LAP2. Journal of Clinical Oncology. 2009;**27**(32):5331-5336. DOI: 10.1200/JCO.2009.22.3248. Epub 2009 Oct 5

[9] Sanchez BR, Mohr CJ, Morton JM, Safadi BY, Alami RS, Curet MJ. Comparison of totally robotic laparoscopic Roux-en-Y gastric bypass and traditional laparoscopic Roux-en-Y gastric bypass. Surgery for Obesity and Related Diseases. 2005;**1**(6):549-554. DOI: 10.1016/j.soard.2005.08.008

[10] Vilallonga R, Fort JM, Caubet E, Gonzalez O, Armengol M. Robotic sleeve gastrectomy versus laparoscopic sleeve gastrectomy: A comparative study with 200 patients. Obesity Surgery. 2013;**23**(10):1501-1507. DOI: 10.1007/s11695-013-1039-3

[11] Scheib SA, Tanner E 3rd, Green IC, Fader AN. Laparoscopy in the morbidly obese: Physiologic considerations and surgical techniques to optimize success. Journal of Minimally Invasive Gynecology. 2014;**21**(2):182-195. DOI: 10.1016/j.jmig.2013.09.009. Epub 2013 Oct 4

[12] Schorge JO. Minimally invasive surgery in morbidly obese women. Obstetrics and Gynecology. 2020;**135**(1):199-210. DOI: 10.1097/AOG.0000000000003588

[13] Mokdad AH, Ford ES, Bowman BA, Dietz WH, Vinicor F, Bales VS, et al. Prevalence of obesity, diabetes, and obesity-related health risk factors, 2001. Journal of the American Medical Association. 2003;**289**(1):76-79. DOI: 10.1001/jama.289.1.76

[14] Lavie CJ, Milani RV, Ventura HO. Obesity and cardiovascular disease: Risk factor, paradox, and impact of weight loss. Journal of the American College of Cardiology. 2009;**53**(21): 1925-1932. DOI: 10.1016/j.jacc.2008.12.068

[15] Lamvu G et al. Obesity: Physiologic changes and challenges during laparoscopy. American Journal of Obstetrics and Gynecology. 2004; **191**(2):669-674

[16] Afors K et al. Obesity in laparoscopic surgery. Best Practice & Research Clinical Obstetrics & Gynaecology. 2015;**29**(4):554-564

[17] Nguyen NT, Wolfe BM. The physiologic effects of pneumo peritoneum in the morbidly obese. Annals of Surgery. 2005;**241**(2):219

[18] Dixon AE, Peters U. The effect of obesity on lung function. Expert Review of Respiratory Medicine. 2018;**12**(9):755-767. DOI: 10.1080/17476348.2018.1506331. Epub 2018 Aug 14

[19] Saliman JA, Benditt JO, Flum DR, Oelschlager BK, Dellinger EP, Goss CH. Pulmonary function in the morbidly obese. Surgery for Obesity and Related Diseases. 2008;**4**(5):632-9; discussion 639. DOI: 10.1016/j.soard.2008.06.010. Epub 2008 Jul 17

[20] Biring MS, Lewis MI, Liu JT, Mohsenifar Z. Pulmonary physiologic changes of morbid obesity. The American Journal of the Medical Sciences. 1999;**318**(5):293-297. DOI: 10.1097/00000441-199911000-00002

[21] Zavorsky GS et al. Waist-to-hip ratio is associated with pulmonary gas exchange in the morbidly obese. Chest. 2007;**131**(2):362-367

[22] Sprung J et al. The impact of morbid obesity, pneumoperitoneum, and posture on respiratory system mechanics and oxygenation during laparoscopy. Anesthesia & Analgesia. 2002;**94**(5):1345-1350

[23] Rahn DD, Mamik MM, Sanses TVD, Matteson KA, Aschkenazi SO, Washington BB, et al. Society of Gynecologic Surgeons Systematic Review GroupVenous thromboembolism prophylaxis in gynecologic surgery: A systematic review. Obstetrics and Gynecology. 2011;**118**(5):1111-1125. DOI: 10.1097/AOG.0b013e318232a394

[24] Kearon C, Akl EA, Comerota AJ, Prandoni P, Bounameaux H, Goldhaber SZ, et al. Antithrombotic therapy for VTE disease: Antithrombotic Therapy and Prevention of Thrombosis, 9th ed: American College of Chest Physicians Evidence-Based Clinical Practice Guidelines. Chest. 2012;**141**(Suppl. 2):e419S-e496S. DOI: 10.1378/chest.11-2301. Erratum in: Chest 2012;142(6):1698-1704

[25] ACOG practice bulletin no. 104: Antibiotic prophylaxis for gynecologic procedures. Obstetrics and Gynecology. 2009;**113**(5):1180-1189. DOI: 10.1097/AOG.0b013e3181a6d011

[26] Tinelli A. Laparoscopic Entry: Traditional Methods, New Insights and Novel Approaches. London, UK: Springer; 2012

[27] Schauer PR, Ikramuddin S, Hamad G, Eid GM, Mattar S, Cottam D, et al. Laparoscopic gastric bypass surgery: Current technique. Journal of Laparoendoscopic & Advanced Surgical Techniques. Part A. 2003;**13**(4):229-239. DOI: 10.1089/109264203322333557

[28] Lundborg G, Dahlin LB. Anatomy, function, and pathophysiology of peripheral nerves and nerve compression. Hand Clinics. 1996;**12**(2):185-193

[29] Louie M, Toubia T, Schiff LD. Considerations for minimally invasive gynecologic surgery in obese patients. Current Opinion in Obstetrics & Gynecology. 2016;**28**(4):283-289. DOI: 10.1097/GCO.0000000000000287

[30] Coppieters MW. Shoulder restraints as a potential cause for stretch

neuropathies: Biomechanical support for the impact of shoulder girdle depression and arm abduction on nerve strain. Anesthesiology. 2006;**104**(6): 1351-1352. DOI: 10.1097/00000542-200606000-00050

[31] Stany MP, Winter WE 3rd, Dainty L, Lockrow E, Carlson JW. Laparoscopic exposure in obese high-risk patients with mechanical displacement of the abdominal wall. Obstetrics and Gynecology. 2004;**103**(2):383-386. DOI: 10.1097/01.AOG.0000110543.14290.35

[32] Hurd WW, Bude RO, DeLancey JO, Pearl ML. The relationship of the umbilicus to the aortic bifurcation: Implications for laparoscopic technique. Obstetrics and Gynecology. 1992;**80**(1): 48-51

[33] Blikkendaal MD et al. Hysterectomy in very obese and morbidly obese patients: A systematic review with cumulative analysis of comparative studies. Archives of Gynecology and Obstetrics. 2015;**292**(4):723-738

[34] Committee on Gynecologic Practice. "Committee opinion no. 619: Gynecologic surgery in the obese woman.". Obstetrics and Gynecology. 2015;**125**(1):274-278

[35] El-Achi V et al. Robotic versus laparoscopic hysterectomy in morbidly obese women for endometrial cancer. Journal of Robotic Surgery. 2021; **15**(3):483-487

[36] Cusimano MC et al. Laparoscopic and robotic hysterectomy in endometrial cancer patients with obesity: A systematic review and meta-analysis of conversions and complications. American Journal of Obstetrics and Gynecology. 2019; **221**(5):410-428

[37] Gala RB et al. Systematic review of robotic surgery in gynecology: Robotic techniques compared with laparoscopy and laparotomy. Journal of Minimally Invasive Gynecology. 2014;**21**(3): 353-361

[38] Albright BB et al. Robotic versus laparoscopic hysterectomy for benign disease: A systematic review and meta-analysis of randomized trials. Journal of Minimally Invasive Gynecology. 2016;**23**(1):18-27

[39] Gossner G, Goldman N. Robotic surgery in the obese gynecologic patient. Clinical Obstetrics and Gynecology. 2011;**54**(3):420-430

[40] Hackethal A et al. Consideration for safe and effective gynaecological laparoscopy in the obese patient. Archives of Gynecology and Obstetrics. 2015;**292**(1):135-141

[41] Uccella S et al. Laparoscopic vs transvaginal cuff closure after total laparoscopic hysterectomy: A randomized trial by the Italian Society of Gynecologic Endoscopy. American Journal of Obstetrics and Gynecology. 2018;**218**(5):500-5e1

[42] Wilcox A, Luciano D, Morosky C. Vaginal Cuff Dehiscence. Topics in Obstetrics & Gynecology. 2020;**40**(13): 1-5

Chapter 5

Bleeding after Hysterectomy: Recommendations and What to Expect

Eugen Ancuța, Radu Zamfir, Gabriel Martinescu, Eduard Crauciuc, Dumitru Sofroni, Larisa Sofroni, Lilian Guțu, Codrina Ancuța and Dragoș Valentin Crauciuc

Abstract

Bleeding after gynecological surgery remains an infrequent life-threatening complication, demanding appropriate medical and surgical management. Classified as early/"reactionary" and delayed/secondary, unexpected postoperative hemorrhage may arise regardless of the route or subtype of hysterectomy. Timely recognition and prompt intervention to arrest bleeding are essential strategies for the suitable outcome of the patient. The present chapter presents an overview on different aspects of bleeding after hysterectomy such as incidence rate, risk factors, mechanisms, and management techniques aiming to expand knowledge and skills in recognizing and treating this unpredicted potentially serious problem. Furthermore, we intend to offer a guide toward standardizing treatment practice across bleeding issues following hysterectomy considering clear recommendations and algorithms.

Keywords: post-surgery bleeding, hysterectomy, reactionary hemorrhage, secondary post-hysterectomy hemorrhage, management

1. Introduction

Considered the second most commonly performed operation after cesarean section worldwide, hysterectomy may be classified as abdominal (laparotomy, laparoscopy, or robotic assistance) and vaginal (via an incision through the superior part of the vagina).

The most common indications for hysterectomy are benign conditions such as uterine fibroids, endometriosis, genital prolapse, pelvic pain, heavy menstrual bleeding, but the technique is also used for gynecological malignancy (usually ovarian, uterine, or cervical) and risk-reducing surgery (in cases of BRCA 1 or 2 mutations or Lynch syndrome) [1–4].

Actually, there are three types of hysterectomy—total hysterectomy (the uterus and cervix are removed), subtotal or partial hysterectomy (the uterus is removed, but the cervix is left in place), and total hysterectomy with bilateral salpingo-oophorectomy (uterus, fallopian tubes, ovaries, and cervix are removed) [1–4]. The term radical hysterectomy (removal of the uterus, cervix, parametrium, vaginal cuff, and fallopian tubes) is used to describe a wide range of procedures universally applicable

IntechOpen

to cervical cancer. However, the degree of radicality clearly depends on preoperative estimation of tumor location, surgical margins and the risk of occult lymphatic spread. Moreover, the ovaries may or may not be removed according to the patient age [1–4]. In addition, supracervical hysterectomy is sometimes preferred to diminish the intraoperative complications and surgical times, as well as to limit the possibility of lower urinary tract issues and maintain normal sexual function [1–4].

The best route for hysterectomy is multifactorial, depending not only on the surgeon's skills and patient safety (minimally invasive procedures as vaginal, laparoscopic, laparoscopic-assisted, and robotic-assisted hysterectomies) but also on economic reasons [1–4].

Hemorrhage after hysterectomy is recognized as an occasional life-threatening complication in modern gynecological surgery, assuming appropriate medical and surgical management [2–9].

Classified as "reactionary" (postoperative bleeding within the first 24 hours following surgery) and secondary (bleeding occurring in the interval 3–22 days after surgery), unexpected hemorrhage may arise regardless of the route or subtype of hysterectomy [5, 6, 9]. Early recognition and prompt intervention (reoperation or arterial embolization) to arrest bleeding are essential strategies for the suitable outcome of the patient [2–10].

While the role of risk factors for "reactionary" hemorrhage is emerging and critical for a correct assessment of the patient, operative laparoscopy is still ideal to treat hemorrhage after vaginal hysterectomy, laparoscopic hysterectomy, laparoscopic-assisted vaginal hysterectomy, and laparotomy being necessary only in selected cases [2–4, 6, 9].

Secondary hemorrhage presents with varying degrees of severity and tends to be more common after laparoscopic hysterectomy, especially total laparoscopic hysterectomy than after the other hysterectomy approaches [5, 9]. Factors potentially responsible are vaginal vault infection, vault hematoma, a poor surgical technique including excessive thermal injury by electrocoagulation, and early resumption of physical activity, large uterus size, excessive use of an energy source for the uterine artery, and culdotomy [2–5, 7, 9, 10].

Ultimately, the management of secondary hemorrhage is challenging and involves diverse approaches based on the exact cause of bleeding, comprising vaginal packing with or without vault suturing, laparoscopic coagulation of the uterine artery if the source of bleeding could not be identified vaginally or arterial embolization [6, 9, 10].

Because of elective gynecologic surgery, we encourage selective patients to donate their own blood before surgery [6, 11]. Several definitions are actually used:

- autologous blood transfusion, when is done with the patient's own blood; blood is stored and can be transfused during surgery;
- homologous transfusion or transfusion from another woman;
- parachute pack or umbrella pack is a useful tool for pelvic bleeding after pelvic exenteration;
- peanut dissector; this tool is indicated for blunt pressure dissection of small places;
- total blood volume; estimated blood volume of total body weight is 8% or 4.5–5.0 liters in the average women. When intraoperative blood loss exceeds 15% of the

blood volume, blood transfusion must be taken into consideration in combating hypovolemic shock. About 15% of an adult blood volume can be calculated by amplification a patient's weight in kg 10 times. The usual method of performing abdominal hysterectomy involved the use of clamps or forceps on vessels.

The present chapter will give an overview on different aspects of bleeding after hysterectomy such as incidence rate, risk factors, mechanisms, and management techniques aiming to expand our knowledge and skills in recognizing and treating this unexpected potentially serious complication. Furthermore, we intend to offer a guide toward standardizing treatment practice across bleeding issues following hysterectomy considering clear recommendations and algorithms.

2. Postoperative bleeding: Current trends/concepts

Postoperative hemorrhage represents a significant potential complication of contemporary gynecological surgery. Despite normal hemostasis, appropriate/suitable surgical technique and close monitoring, postoperative bleeding may occur, leading to the different clinical and operative scenarios and challenging even the most experienced operative team [2–4, 9, 11, 12].

2.1 Subtypes, incidence rate, location, predisposing factors, and complications

2.1.1 Postoperative bleeding subtypes

Based on their timing to surgery, two main subtypes of postoperative hemorrhage are actually recognized [5–9]:

- *subtype 1, early or reactionary postoperative gynecological hemorrhage* where bleeding happens within the first 24 hours following surgery, commonly within the first 4–6 hours postoperative; early bleeding in modern gynecological surgery is reported irrespective of the route of intervention [6, 9];

- *subtype 2, delayed or secondary postoperative bleeding* that develops in the interval 3–22 days after the surgery [5, 9]; secondary hemorrhage is rare and may arise more often after total laparoscopic hysterectomy than after other hysterectomy approaches [5].

2.1.2 Incidence rate of postoperative bleeding

Although the incidence of postoperative hemorrhage basically varies according to surgery, the difference between abdominal, laparoscopic, and vaginal hysterectomy remains statistically insignificant [5–7]. Indeed, some authors postulate that postoperative bleeding occurs more frequently after abdominal and laparoscopic than after vaginal hysterectomy, but overall, the incidence of hemorrhagic events after a hysterectomy varies from 0.2 to 3.1%, irrespective of surgical route [5–8, 10, 13, 14].

On the other hand, the true frequency of delayed bleeding complications is still unknown, although the consequences can be particularly significant in women undergoing outpatient surgery [5–8, 10, 13, 14]. Paul et al. reported an overall cumulative incidence of secondary hemorrhage after a total laparoscopic hysterectomy of 1.3% [5]. Although secondary hemorrhage is rare, it is more often reported after total laparoscopic hysterectomy than after other hysterectomy approaches [5–8, 10, 13, 14].

Table 1 summarizes data on the incidence of postoperative hemorrhage reported by several authors.

2.1.3 Location and source of bleeding

Hemorrhage is responsible for about half of the postoperative complications following gynecological surgery, ranging from persistent venous oozing to massive blood loss from injury to retroperitoneal vessels [5–7, 12, 13].

Main bleeding sites comprise the anterior abdominal wall (both the suprapubic and the umbilical incision), the vaginal cuff (after laparoscopic hysterectomy and laparoscopic-assisted vaginal hysterectomy), and intraabdominal bleeding. Abdominal wall vessel injury occurs with increasing frequency, as the practice of laparoscopic surgery becomes wider and trocars become sharper [2–4, 7, 9].

The source of bleeding in secondary hemorrhage can be the uterine vessels or descending cervical/vaginal vessels; occasionally, uterine artery pseudoaneurysm can cause delayed heavy vaginal bleeding after laparoscopic hysterectomy [2–4, 7, 9]; additionally, the technique of vaginal vault closure may also contribute to the occurrence of secondary hemorrhage [5, 9].

Postoperative pelvic hematoma emerging after gynecological surgery may generate serious morbidity and impaired quality of life if large, infected, or incompletely

Authors	Type of study, no of cases	Incidence postoperative hemorrhage
Makinen et al. [15]	• Large-scale observational study • 10 110 hysterectomies: 5875 AH, 1801 VH, 2434 LH	• The most severe type of hemorrhagic events • Occurred in 2.1%, 3.1%, and 2.7% in the AH, VH and LH group, respectively
Wilke et al. [13]	• Secondary hemorrhage following VH, L-AVH • 1391 cases	• The overall incidence of hemorrhage after VH or LAVH was 1.2% (17 of 1319); • Over the 5-year period, it decreased from 2.4% (five of 209) to 0.6% (two of 315) • The incidence of secondary hemorrhage was 0.23% after VH and LH
Holub and Jabor [7]	• 1226 patients underwent VH or LH for benign or malignant female pelvic diseases between January 1997 and December 2001 • Retrospective analysis	• The overall incidence of postoperative bleeding after LH or VH was 0.85% over a period of 5 years. • During the same period, the incidence of postoperative bleeding ranged from 2/183 (1.1%) in 1997 to 1/231 (0.43%) in 2001 • The frequency of bleeding was 0.93% following LH and 0.71% following VH • 0.17% of secondary hemorrhage after LH and VH
Erian et al. [6]	719 patients between November 1990 and March 2007: 476 VH, 243 LH	• 0.6% in the VH and 1.2% in the LH group
Paul et al. [5]	• 1613 total LH between January 2004 and April 2012 • 21 patients had secondary hemorrhage after hysterectomy	• The overall cumulative incidence of secondary hemorrhage after total laparoscopic hysterectomy was 1.3%

**AH, abdominal hysterectomy; LH, laparoscopic hysterectomy; VH, vaginal hysterectomy; L-AVH, laparoscopic-assisted vaginal hysterectomy.*

Table 1.
*Incidence of postoperative hemorrhage in gynecological surgery.**

resolved hematoma or hematoma with residual fibrosis and persistent pain [2–4, 9]. It usually develops above the vaginal vault, along the pelvic side-wall, retroperitoneal, in the paravesical space, in the abdominal wall as well as in the ischiorectal fossa and vulva [9]. According to its location, postsurgical hematoma may be recognized at routine abdominal and/or pelvic examinations in women with outstanding postoperative discomfort and unexpected anemia, but a definitive diagnosis can only be made by ultrasound or CT scan [5]. A simple or CT/ultrasound-guided or through abdominal incision drainage is commonly required to address the pelvic hematoma issue [2–4, 9].

Postoperative hemorrhage can result from failure to control vascular injury during surgery. Accurate clamp placement, gentle handling of tissues, and the accuracy of dissection are all important and contribute to maximum efficiency with minimum blood loss and minimum tissue damage when abdominal hysterectomy is performed [9].

The electrosurgical instrument can be used for a precise incision of the abdominal wall with minimal tissue injury. By holding the electrode close to the tissue or touching the metal clamp and pressing the coagulation button, superficial coagulation can be achieved [2–4, 9].

2.1.4 Predisposing factors

Intra- and post-operative bleeding generally develops in younger women or those with a more vascular pelvis who underwent a hysterectomy, especially laparoscopic hysterectomy in the presence of fibroids [6, 16].

Possible rationales for secondary hemorrhage comprise a bleeding vessel missed at the end of the procedure, effects of pneumoperitoneum, Trendelenburg position, low intraoperative pressure, wearing off the effect of vasopressin, subacute infection, postoperative analgesia, as well as bleeding disorders [2–5, 7, 9].

Other potential factors accounting for delayed postsurgical bleeding are vaginal vault infection, vault hematoma, poor surgical technique with excessive thermal injury by electrocoagulation, and early resumption of physical activity [5, 7, 9]. A large-sized uterus, high vascularity, large-sized vessels, excessive use of an energy source for the uterine artery, and culdotomy also play a role in this hemorrhagic event [5, 7, 9].

2.1.5 Complications of bleeding

Most of the complications during or after hysterectomy are preventable or treatable. Other complications may exist as medical conditions before hysterectomy but are worsened during surgery, especially if not managed as part of holistic woman's care.

Complications after surgery include [2–4, 9, 12]:

- *hemorrhage*; occurs more often after laparoscopic hysterectomy as compared to vaginal surgery;

- *infections*; occur more often after vaginal hysterectomy than keyhole surgery;

- *damage to internal organs* such as bowel or urinary tract; the injury may occur to the ureter, bladder, or rectum and complications include incontinence, the urgency of urination, and infections;

- *vaginal cuff dehiscence;* is more commonly reported in laparoscopic hysterectomy as compared to laparoscopic assisted procedures or vaginal hysterectomy;

- *anesthetic complications*; smoking, obesity, and heart/lung infections are the most common causes of anesthetic complications;
- *ovarian failure*; interruption to ovarian blood supply following removal of the uterus may precipitate the symptoms of menopause and lead to osteoporosis and ischemic heart disease;
- *low libido*; the removal of the uterus may lead to less sexual enjoyment due to the loss of uterine contractions;
- *venous thromboembolism*; prophylactic anticoagulants are associated with a lowering of the risk for such events;
- *depression*; most of the women complain of feeling depressed because they have lost an important part of them.

In Romania, the mortality rate following a hysterectomy is very low.

Contemporary management of surgical interventions includes postoperative bleeding and the possibility of blood transfusion with risks of HIV transmission (in 1.9 million cases), the transmission of hepatitis B (one in every 180.000 cases), or a febrile reaction to transfusion (1% cases) [2]. Most experts recommend acute normovolemic hemodilution and cell salvage in women undergoing hysterectomy section who will not accept blood products.

Hypovolemic shock can occur after major bleeding as a direct result of uncontrolled hemorrhage. Depending on the total blood volume lost, hypovolemic shock may be divided into four classes: I (< 75 mL or 15%), II (750–1500 mL, or 15–30%), III (1500–2000 mL or 30–40%) and IV (>2000 mL or > 40%) [6].

The clinical manifestations of class I hypovolemia are not measurable and compensatory mechanisms restore plasma volume within a day. In class II hypovolemia, tachycardia is the most frequent clinical finding as a result of inadequate circulatory volume. The distinction between class I and II hypovolemic shock is made by recording blood pressure and pulse in the standing, sitting, or reclining position. Postural hypotension is observed as result of cardiac failure. Compensatory mechanisms begin to fail with the class III hypovolemic shock. This results in an increase in the arterial and venous oxygen difference with classic signs including worked tachycardia, tachypnea, oliguria, and cold skin. With the class IV hypovolemic shock, a patient's survival depends on rapid transfusion of blood and immediate surgical intervention before cardiovascular collapse and death or organ system failure.

After initial resuscitative measures are instituted, it is highly recommended for patients to be carried out in a critical care unit. Use of sympathomimetic agents after sufficient hydration and vasodilator is normally preferred in the management of patients with hemorrhagic shock who have arterial pressure higher than 70 mm Hg.

Once restoration of the intravascular volume has been completed, it is important to reassess the patient's response to blood transfusion when managing women with severe blood loss, especially in those patients who have pulmonary edema, myocardial infarction, or congestive heart failure [12].

Transfusion for patients with hemoglobin of 8–10 mg/dL is no longer recommended.

When major surgery is anticipated and transfusion is massive, platelets in addition to packed cell transfusion are required. It is recommended that cryoprecipitate be reserved for patients with deficiencies in von Willebrand factor, factor VIII, and fibrinogen factor XIII.

2.2 Management of postoperative hemorrhage

Recognized as an uncommon complication of hysterectomy, postoperative hemorrhage represents a true challenge in routine practice [8]; irrespective of the procedure, a close follow-up of the patient in a high-dependency unit is indicated in order to exclude recurrence of bleeding [6, 7].

The key to successful management is timely intervention meaning prompt diagnosis, urgent resuscitation if necessary and rapid decision for either arterial embolization or reoperation according to the severity of bleeding and the hemodynamic stability of the patient. Both techniques are highly effective to control bleeding; nevertheless, if the patient is hemodynamically unstable or of the interval since surgery is under 24 hours suggesting rapid hemorrhage, the emergency return to the operating theater to arrest the bleeding is preferred [6, 7, 9].

Current options for managing hemorrhage include [6, 7, 9]:

- every patient should be carefully monitored postoperatively for signs of bleeding (hypotension, tachycardia, tachypnea, abdominal distension);

- ultrasound can confirm intraperitoneal bleeding; more ways to determine intraabdominal hemorrhage include abdominal and pelvic CT scan; a routine coagulation profile should be done immediately for the patient with a rapid pulse, low blood pressure, and/or low urine output. The surgeon must take charge of the problem and execute the technical steps necessary to treat hemorrhagic shock in the operating room. Intraperitoneal bleeding can be hidden by incisional pain and analgesic medications. Despite adequate dissection, a small vessel may bleed or the suture may cut through tissue. Skeletonized vessels and small sutures should be used for significantly reducing the incidence of postoperative hemorrhage. Venous bleeding can be more life-threatening than arterial hemorrhage which can be clearly seen and controlled with fast small sutures or clamps.

- the presence of unexpected drop in hematocrit or hemoglobin postoperatively.

A simplified algorithm to describe steps after gynecological surgery and potential post-surgery bleeding is provided in **Figure 1**.

A closer look at the holistic management of postoperative blood should also underpin the following [9]:

- to assess blood value and coagulation mechanisms;

- to identify changes in the coagulation components, and to initiate replacement therapy in order to achieve adequate hemostasis. In assessing the patient's coagulation status, it is very important to avoid such a situation known as the trauma triad of death consisting of—hypothermia, metabolic acidosis, and coagulopathy. In some patients with benign disease, blood transfusion is rarely indicated. Experience has shown that blood transfusion may be significant in women with malignant disease;

- to establish the therapeutic strategy by measuring the level of prothrombin time < 14 sec, activated partial thromboplastin time (aptt) < 40 sec, fibrinogen >100 mg/dL, platelets >80 × 10^3 mL.

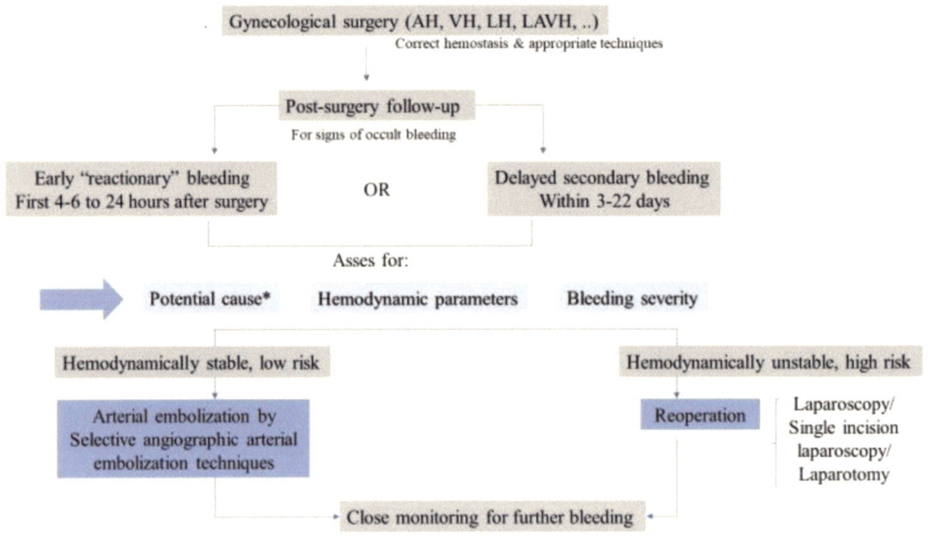

Figure 1.
A simplified algorithm of post-surgery bleeding approach.

2.2.1 Reoperation

In hemodynamically unstable women (rapid pulse, falling blood pressure, with or without renal impairment) or if the bleeding occurs shortly in post-surgery (the so-called reactionary hemorrhage), it is desirable to return to the operating room [5–9].

A preoperative abdominal and pelvic ultrasound or CT scan is routinely required to visualize the source of bleeding as being intra- or retro-peritoneal, as well as adequate local examination without or under anesthesia. Moreover, the operative procedure should be mentally revised to identify any potential bleeding issue [9].

Surgical revision for postoperative bleeding may be performed transvaginally, laparoscopically, or both [5–9, 13, 14].

Postoperative hemorrhage from the vaginal vault recurrently originates from the vaginal artery in the lateral vaginal fornix or from one of its branches, since the lateral vaginal angle which includes the vaginal artery may not be accurately protected or turn into disligated [9, 13, 14]. Excessive vaginal bleeding needs to be objectively measured; since the vagina is a distensible organ, clots obstructing the vaginal introitus may lead to a large amount of blood accumulating and distending the vagina, subsequently covering the true significance of hemorrhage [9, 13, 14]. Vaginal bleeding can be controlled by clamping and ligating the bleeding point as well as by delayed-absorbable transfixion suturing of the vaginal mucosa and paravaginal tissue [9, 13, 14]. If such techniques are not enough or bleeding vessels have retracted, other tactics should be intended [8].

When no noticeable vaginal source, bleeding after abdominal or vaginal hysterectomy is traditionally treated by laparotomy or laparoscopy [7, 9]. While laparotomy is recommended in cases of intraperitoneal bleeding or unsuccessful conservative transvaginal treatment, operative laparoscopy is clearly indicated if the source of bleeding cannot be identified by the means of vaginal examination and/or if an intraabdominal bleeding source is suspected [7, 9, 13].

2.2.2 Laparotomy

Post-surgery bleeding requires laparotomy in two situations.

Firstly, if the surgical hemostasis cannot be achieved transvaginally, laparotomy may be necessary [9].

Secondly, if the patient underwent an abdominal hysterectomy, the incision should be reopened, succeeding the following steps (i) clots and blood evacuation from the abdomen and pelvic area; (ii) searching of the potential bleeding sites, commencing with the most expected places; (iii) ligating, suturing, or clipping of the identified bleeding sites; (iv) verifying the ureteral integrity as high risk of ureteral damage during reoperation; and (v) closing second time after a completely dry abdomen and pelvis [9].

2.2.3 Laparoscopy

The laparoscopic approach to postoperative bleeding following laparoscopic hysterectomy, vaginal hysterectomy, or laparoscopic-assisted vaginal hysterectomy is an attractive alternative to the abdominal surgical approach in the majority of patients [6, 7, 9, 13]. The procedure can be used to adequately evaluate the pelvis and the abdominal wall, which is occasionally the source of hemorrhage after laparoscopic hysterectomy. Moreover, whether the bleeding is from the abdominal wall, the surgical pedicles, or the vaginal cuff, it can be managed laparoscopically [8, 9]. Evidently, hemostasis can be more easily obtained in laparoscopic surgery because of magnification, close inspection, routine use of suction irrigation, and bipolar coagulation [7, 9]. Besides, bipolar coagulation, a Foley catheter introduced in the port-site bleeding, or a collagen-fibrin agent can be used to achieve local hemostasis during laparoscopy [7, 9].

Following laparoscopic irrigation/suction using Ringer's solution to clear the operative field, a combination of laparoscopic suturing using absorbable suture material and laparoscopic bipolar coagulation is commonly recommended [6, 8, 9]. Also, electrosurgery is effective in controlling bleeding during laparoscopic surgery. Furthermore, different forms of fibrin adhesive are tested in gynecologic open surgery in order to stop oozing hemorrhages after primary hemostatic treatment with a high efficacy rate (98%) [6]. Holub and Kliment reported successful treatment of hemorrhage from damaged tissue near important pelvic structures using the laparoscope to apply collagen fleece combined with fibrin glue [7, 17].

To avoid further risk of injury to the abdominal wall and to improve the recovery time from surgery, *single incision laparoscopic surgery* is a viable option for the management of hemorrhage, particularly for those patients whose original surgery was accomplished via single incision laparoscopic surgery. Curlin et al. reported a case where single incision laparoscopy was used to manage postoperative hemorrhage after total laparoscopic hysterectomy with right salpingectomy and left salpingo-oophorectomy [8].

2.3 Arterial embolization

Conversely, if the patient is reasonably stable and there is not abrupt early bleeding (based on the volume of blood in the abdomen or retroperitoneal space as estimated by ultrasound and the time from surgery), it seems realistic to try to identify the bleeding artery and embolize it by transcatheter interventional radiological techniques [2–4, 9, 10].

Arterial embolization remains an important minimally invasive option for the management of delayed postoperative hemorrhage [2–4, 8, 9, 18]. Transcatheter arterial embolization has been shown to be an effective tool for the management of postoperative hemorrhage after gynecologic laparoscopy, but also after abdominal and vaginal hysterectomy [8, 9]. Selective angiographic arterial embolization is a quite simple and safe procedure with a clinical success rate up to 90% in routine practice and usually a low complication rate less than 10%, including a mild postembolization syndrome with pain, fever, high leucocyte count related to vascular thrombosis and tissue necrosis [8, 9]. Bladder necrosis, vesicovaginal fistula, neuropathies as well as renal toxicity are uncommon, isolated side effects [9].

Arterial embolization technique comprises the following main steps—(i) identification of the site of bleeding by angiofluoroscopy if more than 2–3 mL/min bleeding rate; (ii) percutaneous catheterization of the femoral artery or, uncommonly, brachial artery under local anesthesia with retrograde direct access to the hypogastric artery; (iii) canulation of the hypogastric artery or specific collateral vessel if appropriate; (iv) injection of the embolization material under angiographic observation (metal coins, autologous clot, small pieces of gelfoam, small silastic spheres, subcutaneous tissue, or other hemostatic materials; (v) repeat angiography to demonstrate the occlusion of the bleeding vessel; (vi) remove of the catheter followed by careful monitoring for further bleeding [8–10].

Although second surgery is often the initial choice for postoperative hemorrhage, for a patient who is hemodynamically stable but is experiencing postoperative hemorrhage, transcatheter arterial embolization is a welcome alternative to a second surgery [8, 9]. However, if rapid access to interventional radiology is not available or if transcatheter arterial embolization is unsuccessful, laparoscopy can still be considered [8, 9]. Besides, a potential advantage of surgical management of postoperative hemorrhage over transcatheter arterial embolization is the ability to evacuate the hemoperitoneum, which may decrease postoperative pain, the risk of infection, and the risk of ileus [8, 9].

3. Recommendations for managing postoperative bleeding in gynecological surgery

It is typical to expect some bleeding after hysterectomy in the 6–8 weeks following the procedure; the discharge may be red, brown, or pink. Bleeding should steadily decrease in the days and weeks following the surgery and should never be excessive at any point of recovery [18]. The exception is menstruation in women who have undergone a subtotal hysterectomy [18, 19]. In case of bleeding after hysterectomy, it is more likely to be of some pathologic cause instead of menstruation which needs to be ruled out [19].

However, a sudden and significant increase in bleeding during recovery should be considered abnormal. Points of concern comprise but are not limited to—bright red vaginal bleeding (indicating active bleed), temperature over 100.4°F, severe nausea or vomiting, increasing pelvic pain, a local complication such as redness, swelling, or drainage at the incision site as well as difficulty in urinating or pain with urination suggesting either an infection or a neurogenic bladder [18].

Delayed vaginal hemorrhage after laparoscopic supracervical hysterectomy usually requires emergent reoperation. Several studies have described continued cyclical bleeding from the cervical stump after supracervical hysterectomy in 0–25% of cases [20].

Effective interventions addressing hemorrhage after hysterectomy are needed to reduce women's mortality worldwide.

DOI: http://dx.doi.org/10.5772/intechopen.101384

3.1 Recommendations

a. *Counseling*

Prior to hysterectomy, these women should be offered specific counseling and have a prospective plan for the management of their disease, developed by gynecologists of how their condition and hysterectomy interact. Prehysterectomy counseling services starting for all women planning this surgical intervention are a key part of hospital services and should be an integral part of the local health services network. They could be provided by general practitioners or specialist clinicians or surgeons, all of whom should be suitably trained or may require different management or specialized services before hysterectomy. There are special circumstances as congenital or acquired coagulation disorders that should be considered to evaluate by a thorough history and lab tests.

b. Professional interpretation services for women who do not speak English.

It is not clear how much the specific medical terminology is conveyed to the patient. Healthcare providers have to invest in technology, security, specialists, and translators to ensure healthcare becomes world-class. Medical tourism is growing each year. Romania provides the highest quality healthcare at the lowest price. Also, the cost of hysterectomy in Romania is lower than the same treatment in UK or UE. In developed countries as the USA, UE countries or Canada patients have to wait a long time for major surgeries. The cost involved in treating a patient depends upon factors like—type of hysterectomy needed, hospital and physician selected for it, and duration of staying.

c. Communication and referrals among professionals.

Good communication among professionals is essential. Referral between specialties involved should be rapid. They can use a variety of communication methods including—mobile phone, email, fax, Whatsapp, Instagram, Tik Tok, Facebook, etc. In many cases, junior trainees in the front line did not have proper support and need to have clear guidelines about when to seek senior help.

d. Women with serious medical conditions

They require immediate and appropriate multidisciplinary specialist care; women will require referral to tertiary or specialist medical centers for their preexisting medical or mental conditions before hysterectomy. Conditions that require prehysterectomy counseling and advice include—epilepsy, diabetes, asthma, congenital or known acquired cardiac disease, autoimmune disorders, renal and liver disease, obesity (BMI > 30), severe mental illness, or psychiatric conditions that require a change of medication, HIV infection. Women with potential serious underlying preexisting medical on mental health conditions should be immediately referred to appropriate specialist centers of expertise as soon as their symptoms develop.

e. Clinical training

All clinical staff must undertake regular training for the identification and management of serious disease conditions or potential emergencies or signs and symptoms of potentially life-threatening conditions, circulatory failure, severe hypertension or major hemorrhage, pyrexia >38°C, tachycardia >100 bpm, breathlessness. The local clinicians may be excellent at the management of severely ill women but must also accept written, documented, and audited courses. There should be a well-trained team of doctors for recording and charting investigations performed, obtaining quick results, ensuring that abnormal results are followed up promptly and have resulted in a better outcome.

f. Identifying and managing very sick women with critical illness before, during or after hysterectomy

In very acute situations, a team approach can be very healthful. The management of patients with an acute severe illness with circulatory failure, arterial hypertension, and major hemorrhage requires a team approach and help from the anesthetic and critical care services. There are some healthcare professionals who failed to manage crisis situations outside their immediate area of expertise; therefore, it is crucial to recognize their limitations and to know when and whom to call for another opinion once the patient was admitted to the hospital.

Coagulation factors, hematocrit, serum calcium, glucose, and electrolytes could be assessed every 120 minutes or after 10 U of transfusion; these lab tests are very helpful for the diagnosis of postoperative bleeding.

RCOG guidelines of the responsibilities of the consultant on call should be followed.

Bilateral hypogastric artery ligation can reduce blood loss to a minimum during hysterectomy [9].

Hypotensive anesthesia is also a safe and effective technique in reducing the circulation to the operative field [9].

g. Serious incident and women death reporting

Health professionals, senior or junior, must recognize an act on the signs and symptoms of potentially life-threatening conditions.

The evaluation of such a report must include clinicians from relevant disciplines (including anesthetics) who were not involved with the deaths. This report is recommended to be a requirement in the future.

The identification and act on women's death should be reviewed as a serious incident and disseminated to all health professionals, junior or senior. Women's deaths are generally underreported because of incorrect classification of cause.

Fatal hemorrhage can result from laceration of the external iliac vein or the hypogastric vein where they join together which are at risk of injury when the surgeon dissects between the distal common iliac artery, the psoas muscle, and the area of lumbosacral nerve trunks [9]. These vessels cannot be clamped and ligated with clips or sutures [9].

Dissection around the aorta and vena cava done with inadequate exposure performed in order to remove lymph nodes around them can result in serious hemorrhage. Bleeding usually can be avoided by placing a finger over the laceration and a vascular needle is used to close the laceration from side to side. The same technique may be used for common and external iliac veins [9].

Also, bleeding can occur by dissecting pararectal space and presacral space as well as obturator fossa [9].

h. Pathology

Patient death autopsy must be improved and require more expertise.

DOI: http://dx.doi.org/10.5772/intechopen.101384

In Romania, the number of women death after hysterectomy (death rate) is very small and many of the autopsies reviewed were considered adequate. When an autopsy is needed, the body can be taken to another area for more expert examination. Despite evaluation by many examiners in the different specialties, the final diagnosis could not be resolved because of inadequate clinical data, poor autopsy quality, or the unmanageable nature of some death.

4. Conclusion

The lack of routine observation in the postoperative period or a failure to appreciate blood loss or recognition of abnormal vital signs such as oxygen saturation and respiratory rate can lead to death after hysterectomy. The patient should be evaluated before hysterectomy for risk factors and the medical conditions of the women should be diagnosed by a careful history and lab tests in order to decrease the possibility of hemorrhage.

The risks of blood transfusion, the transmission of HIV or hepatitis B should be discussed before surgical procedure.

The peace of surgical intervention should be governed by good exposure of the tissue, accuracy of dissection, and clamping or suturing the vessels in a precise manner. The skills and experiences of the surgeon without wasting time with unnecessary hesitation or indecision will reduce the risk of uncontrolled hemorrhage after a hysterectomy.

The surgeon should control the life-threatening hemorrhage by judgment, knowledge, and technical skills. The patient's medical history for vital signs, blood loss volume, and levels of coagulation factors will determine how quickly blood transfusion is initiated. Careful postoperative clinical evaluation of the patient by the surgeon and surgical team with abdominal or pelvic ultrasound or CT scanning will help to prevent or minimize significant blood loss after hysterectomy and localize the site of bleeding.

Acknowledgements

No funding was received for this chapter.

Author details

Eugen Ancuța[1*], Radu Zamfir[2], Gabriel Martinescu[3], Eduard Crauciuc[4], Dumitru Sofroni[5], Larisa Sofroni[6], Lilian Guțu[7], Codrina Ancuța[4*] and Dragoș Valentin Crauciuc[4]

1 Research Department, "Elena Doamna" Obstetrics and Gynecology Clinical Hospital, Iași, Romania'

2 Hepatobiliary and Liver Transplant Department, "Fundeni" Clinical Institute, București, Romania

3 "Elena Doamna" Obstetrics and Gynecology Clinical Hospital, Iași, Romania

4 University of Medicine and Pharmacy "Grigore T. Popa", Iasi, Romania

5 University of Medicine and Pharmacy "Nicolae Testemitanu", Chisinau, Republic of Moldova

6 Institute of Oncology, Chisinau, Republic of Moldova

7 Medpark International Hospital, Chisinau, Republic of Moldova

*Address all correspondence to: eugen01ro@yahoo.com and codrina_ancuta@yahoo.com

References

[1] Dawood AS, Elbohoty SB, Abbas AM, Elgergawy AE. Colpotomizer-assisted total abdominal hysterectomy (CATAH Technique): A new technique for uterine removal in benign pathologies. Gynecology and Minimally Invasive Therapy. 2021;**10**(2):109-113

[2] Jones HW III, Hysterectomy A. In: Rock J, Jones H III, editors. TeLinde's Operative Gynecology. 10th ed. Philadelphia: Lippincott Williams & Wilkins, Wolters Kluwer Health; 2008. pp. 727-744

[3] Kovac RS. Vaginal Hysterectomy. In: Rock J, Jones H III, editors. TeLinde's operative Gynecology. 10th ed. Philadelphia: Lippincott Williams & Wilkins, Wolters Kluwer Health; 2008. pp. 744-763

[4] Howarsd F. Laparoscopic Hysterectomy. In: Rock J, Jones H III, editors. TeLinde's Operative Gynecology. 10th ed. Philadelphia: Lippincott Williams & Wilkins, Wolters Kluwer Health; 2008. pp. 763-776

[5] Paul PG, Prathap T, Kaur H, et al. Secondary hemorrhage after total laparoscopic hysterectomy. JSLS. 2014;**18**(3):e2014.00139. DOI: 10.4293/JSLS.2014.00139

[6] Erian M, Mc Laren G, Khalil A. Reactionary hemorrhage in gynecological surgery. JSLS. 2008;**12**(1):81-84

[7] Holub Z, Jabor A. Laparoscopic management of bleeding after laparoscopic or vaginal hysterectomy. JSLS. 2004;**8**(3):235-238

[8] Curlin H, Scheib S. Single incision laparoscopy for the management of postoperative hemorrhage. JSLS. 2012;**16**(3):478-480

[9] Jones HW III, Rock WA Jr. Control of pelvic hemorrhage. In: Rock J, Jones H III, editors. TeLinde's Operative Gynecology. 10th ed. Philadelphia: Lippincott Williams & Wilkins, Wolters Kluwer Health; 2008. pp. 371-394

[10] Takeda A, Koyama K, Mori M, Sakai K, Mitsui T, Nakamura H. Diagnostic computed tomographic angiography and therapeutic emergency transcatheter arterial embolization for management of postoperative hemorrhage after gynecologic laparoscopic surgery. Journal of Minimally Invasive Gynecology. 2008;**15**:332-341

[11] Katz VL. Preoperative counseling and management – patient evaluation, informed consent, infection prophylaxis, avoidance of complications. In: Katz V, Lentz G, Lobo R, Gershenson D, editors. Comprehensive Gynecology. 5th ed. Philadelphia: Mosby Elsevier; 2007

[12] Katz VL. Postoperative counseling and management – fever, respiratory, cardiovascular, thromboembolic, urinary tract, gastrointestinal, wound, operative site, neurologic injury, psychological sequelae. In: Katz V, Lentz G, Lobo R, Gershenson D, editors. Comprehensive Gynecology. 5th ed. Philadelphia: Mosby Elsevier; 2007

[13] Wilke I, Merker A, Schneider A. Laparoscopic treatment of hemorrhage after vaginal hysterectomy or laparoscopically assisted vaginal hysterectomy (LAVH). Surgical Endoscopy. 2001;**15**(10):1144-1146

[14] Yamashita Y, Harada M, Yamamoto H, et al. Transcatheter arterial embolization of obstetric and gynaecologic bleeding: Efficacy and clinical outcome. The British Journal of Radiology. 1994;**67**:530-534

[15] Makinen J, Johansson J, Tomas C, et al. Morbidity of 11 110 hysterectomies by type of approach. Human Reproduction. 2001;**16**:1473-1478

[16] McPherson K, Metcalfe MA, Herbert A, et al. Severe complications of hysterectomy: The VALUE study. BJOG: An International Journal of Obstetrics and Gynaecology. 2004;**111**(7):688-694

[17] Holub Z, Kliment L. The effectiveness of collagen fleece combined with a fibrin glue in hemostasis during laparoscopic surgery. Journal of Gynecologic Surgery. 1999;**15**:185-191

[18] Whitlock J. Bleeding after a hysterectomy. Available from: https://www.verywellhealth.com/bleeding-after-a-hysterectomy-3156906 [Accessed: October 15, 2021]

[19] Lyngdoh BT, Kriplani A, Garg P, et al. Post-hysterectomy menstruation: A rare phenomenon. Archives of Gynecology and Obstetrics. 2010;**281**:307-309. DOI: 10.1007/s00404-009-1173-2

[20] Holloran-Schwartz MB, Potter SJ, Kao MS. Massive delayed vaginal hemorrhage after laparoscopic supracervical hysterectomy. Case report. Case Reports in Obstetrics and Gynecology. 2012;**2012**:871041. DOI: 10.1155/2012/871041

Chapter 6

Surgical Site Infection after Hysterectomy

Catherine W. Chan and Michael L. Nimaroff

Abstract

Surgical site infections (SSIs) are associated with increased morbidity, mortality, and healthcare costs. SSIs are defined as an infection that occurs after surgery in the part of the body where the surgery took place. Approximately 1–4% of hysterectomies are complicated by SSIs, with higher rates reported for abdominal hysterectomy. Over the past decade, there has been an increasing number of minimally invasive hysterectomies, in conjunction with a decrease in abdominal hysterectomies. The reasons behind this trend are multifactorial but are mainly rooted in the well-documented advantages of minimally invasive surgery. Multiple studies have demonstrated a marked decrease in morbidity and mortality with minimally invasive surgeries. Specifically, evidence supports lower rates of SSIs after laparoscopic hysterectomy when compared to abdominal hysterectomy. In fact, the American College of Obstetricians and Gynecologist recommends minimally invasive approaches to hysterectomy whenever feasible. This chapter will review the current literature on surgical site infection (SSI) after hysterectomy for benign indications.

Keywords: infection, hysterectomy

1. Introduction

Hysterectomy is one of the most commonly performed surgeries in the United States. In fact, Merrill et al. reported a 45% lifetime risk of hysterectomy [1] with an overall rate of 5.4 per 1000 women per year. The majority of hysterectomies are performed for benign gynecologic conditions—that is, the presence of fibroids. Other indications include abnormal uterine bleeding, uterovaginal prolapse, and pelvic pain. Hysterectomy can be performed via multiple routes—abdominally, laparoscopically (including robotic approach), or vaginally. Vaginal and laparoscopic procedures are considered minimally invasive surgical approaches based on the ability to avoid a large abdominal incision. These routes of hysterectomy are associated with shortened hospitalization and postoperative recovery when compared to the abdominal approach. As a result, analysis of U.S. surgical data demonstrates evolving practice patterns with an increase in minimally invasive hysterectomies and a decrease in abdominal hysterectomies [2, 3].

The Centers for Disease Control and Prevention defines surgical site infection (SSI) as an infection that occurs after surgery near the surgical site within 30 days following surgery or 90 days where an implant is involved. They can range from superficial infections involving skin, or more serious infections involving tissues underneath the skin, organs, or implanted materials. As such, SSI is classified as superficial, deep, or organ/space. The CDC monitors SSI via the National Healthcare

Safety Network with reported SSI rates of 1.7% and 0.9% after abdominal and vaginal hysterectomy respectively [4].

In a retrospective cohort study of 23,366 patients undergoing laparoscopic and abdominal hysterectomy between the years 2005 and 2011, 783 (3%) developed a surgical site infection. The majority of these were wound infections with approximately ¼ of cases being infections of the organ space which represents 0.7% of the entire cohort [5]. A more recent large cohort study examining patients between the years 2012 and 2015 demonstrated a 2% incidence of postoperative infection after hysterectomy [6]. When stratified between abdominal versus minimally invasive approaches, the incidence of SSI in the abdominal hysterectomy group exceeded 1%, while the incidences in the other groups were 0.2–0.3% [7–9].

It is well known that postoperative infections are associated with increased patient morbidity and mortality, and may result in additional costs, extended hospital stays, and prolonged antibiotic use. On average, patients who had an SSI following hysterectomy incur twice the cost of care of their counterparts who did not have an SSI. In a study examining the clinical and economic burden of surgical site infection following hysterectomy, the highest cost owing to SSI ($19,203; 95% CI 17,260–21,365) was for abdominal hysterectomy. In addition, those who had SSI had a mean length of stay (LOS) that was between three and fivefold the LOS of those who did not have an SSI irrespective of surgical approach [10]. SSI following index surgery is also associated with a significantly greater percentage of hospital readmissions. Surgical site infections after hysterectomy have serious implications on patient care and healthcare as a whole. This chapter will review the current literature on surgical site infection (SSI) after hysterectomy for benign indications and address various methods of prevention and treatment.

2. Route of hysterectomy

There are a variety of factors that influence the route of hysterectomy including informed patient preference, accessibility of the uterus, extent of extrauterine disease, size and shape of the vagina and uterus, concurrent procedures, available hospital technology and support, the nature of the case—whether it is emergent or scheduled, and surgeon training and experience. The American College of Obstetricians and Gynecologists (ACOG) recommends vaginal hysterectomy as the approach of choice whenever feasible [11].

Evidence supports that the vaginal approach is associated with better outcomes when compared with other approaches to hysterectomy. A Cochrane review analyzing 47 randomized control trials with a total of 5,102 women determined that vaginal hysterectomy resulted in quicker return to normal activity when compared to abdominal hysterectomy. There was no difference in satisfaction, quality of life, and surgical complications. Similarly, laparoscopic hysterectomy also resulted in more rapid recovery, fewer febrile episodes, and lower incidence of SSI when compared to the abdominal approach [12]. In this systematic review, there were no advantages of laparoscopic over vaginal hysterectomy. In addition, the laparoscopic approach was associated with longer operating times and increased rates of urinary tract injuries [13]. As a result, a vaginal approach continues to be the preferred route of hysterectomy.

When it is not feasible to perform a vaginal hysterectomy, a surgeon must choose between a laparoscopic or an open abdominal approach. A Cochrane review demonstrated faster return to normal activity, shorter hospital stay, fewer infections, and improved quality of life in patients undergoing laparoscopic versus abdominal hysterectomy. However, operating times were longer with higher rates of lower urinary tract (bladder and ureter) injuries in the laparoscopy group [13].

When stratified by the type of hysterectomy—total laparoscopic hysterectomy (TLH), laparoscopic-assisted vaginal hysterectomy (LAVH), and laparoscopic supracervical hysterectomy (LSCH)—a comparison of the 30-day incidence of deep or organ-space and superficial incisional SSIs in 46,755 women demonstrated a decreased risk of deep or organ-space SSI in the LSCH group compared to the other subtypes [14]. The overall rate of 30-day deep or organ-space SSI was 1.8%. There were no differences in superficial SSI in all groups; however, the rate of deep or organ-space SSI was lower in women who underwent LSCH (0.6%) compared with TLH (1.0%) and LAVH (1.1%).

When stratified into various forms of laparoscopic hysterectomy including robotic hysterectomy, laparoscopic-assisted vaginal hysterectomy, and single-port hysterectomy, the authors concluded that more research was needed to determine if there is in fact, a benefit over conventional laparoscopic approaches. The largest study available on single port laparoscopy in gynecology was a retrospective study from Cleveland Clinic reviewing a total of 908 cases. The authors concluded that single port access was safe and feasible in gynecologic surgery inclusive of both malignant and premalignant conditions with a low rate of adverse outcomes. Perhaps the most prevalent adverse outcome is an increased risk of incisional hernia with a rate of 5.5% [15, 16]. Well-designed studies that compare outcomes of alternative hysterectomy routes (robotic, laparoscopic assisted vaginal, and single-port) are needed to determine if patients may benefit from these other approaches.

Although minimally invasive routes to hysterectomy remain the preferred approach, open abdominal hysterectomy is still an important surgical option for some patients. Open abdominal hysterectomy may become necessary in a variety of clinical scenarios including failure of to maintain a minimally invasive approach.

3. Prevention of SSI

3.1 Preoperative risk factors

Preoperative medical optimization is critically important in risk reduction for SSI prior to hysterectomy. Eliminating particular risk factors for SSI contributes vastly to perioperative care. This includes taking an in-depth medical history, performing a comprehensive physical exam, and addressing the patient's medical comorbidities. Patients should be counseled on modifiable and nonmodifiable risk factors such as smoking status, diabetes stabilization, anatomic anomalies, renal comorbidities, hydrosalpinx, endometrioma, prior laparotomy, and untreated pelvic inflammatory disease (PID) or bacterial vaginosis [17–20]. Optimal diabetes control is critical in preventing postoperative SSI with both spot glucose levels ≤200 mg/dl and hemoglobin A1C levels below 8.5–9.0% [21, 22].

Preoperative screening for genital tract infections is generally not necessary; however, certain types of infections are clinically important prior to hysterectomy. It has been well established that bacterial vaginosis (BV) is associated with an increased risk of postoperative cuff cellulitis and subsequent pelvic abscess formation after hysterectomy [23]. Treatment of BV prior to scheduled hysterectomy will decrease this risk.

3.2 Intraoperative interventions

Practicing safe, high-quality, evidence-based operating room care begins first with accurate identification of the patient, surgical site, and procedure.

In an AAGL white paper, "Enhanced Recovery and Surgical Optimization Protocol for Minimally Invasive Gynecologic Surgery", infection prophylaxis can be achieved via the implementation of SSI prevention bundles [24]. Quality or safety bundles provide a framework for the implementation of evidence-based practices. They have been validated across multiple disciplines to actually decrease SSI [25–28]. The ACOG Council on Patient Safety in Women's Health Care has published a consensus bundle on prevention of SSI prior to gynecologic surgery. This provides a framework for hospitals to develop, implement, and practice evidence-based prevention of SSIs [29].

An example of a hysterectomy bundle is as follows:

Abdominal Hysterectomy
Process Checklists
(Quality Improvement Data Sheet: Not for Medical Record)

Facility Name:		**Date:**	**Scheduled Elective** ☐ **Add-on** ☐ **Emergent** ☐
Procedure Performed:			
Surgeon:		**Admission Location: Inpatient** ☐	**Same Day Admission** ☐
Unit	**Responsibility**	**Action Taken**	**Action Documented**
Same Day Ad mission (SDA)	Pre-Procedure RN	**Pre-operative body wash with 2% or 4% chlorhexidine gluconate (CHG):** 1. Was the body wash done 2 days prior to surgery? 2. Was the body wash done 1 day (night before or morning of surgery) prior to surgery? 3. Was separate sponge used for each body wash? 4. Did patient use fresh linen and fresh towels after body wash? 5. Did patient wear fresh clothing after the body wash? 6. Were CHG wipes used in pre-operative are prior to surgery?	 Yes ☐ No ☐ Yes ☐ No ☐ Yes ☐ No ☐ Yes ☐ No ☐ Yes ☐ No ☐ Yes ☐ No ☐
	Completed by:		(Print Name)
	SDA RN or Pre-Procedure RN	**Temperature - Goal Range 36° - 38°C:** 1. Temperature ≥ 36° C on arrival to SDA? 2. Warming device applied? Identify type: ☐ Bair Paws ☐ Bair Hugger ☐ Other **If temperature is ≥ 36°C, no further temperatures are needed. If ≤ 36°C retake the temperature at 1 hour.** 1 Temperature at 1 hour ≥ 36°C? 2. Surgery is on hold until temperature ≥ 36°C (Elective Only)?	Temperature:________ Yes ☐ No ☐ Yes ☐ No ☐ Temperature:________ Yes ☐ No ☐ N/A ☐ Yes ☐ No ☐ N/A ☐
		Blood glucose (Targeted goal < 200): 1. What is the patient's blood glucose (BS) result in SDA? 2. If > 200 mg/dL was Anesthesia and the Surgeon notified? 3. Surgery on hold until treated and ≤ 200 (Elective Only)?	 BS:____________ Yes ☐ No ☐ N/A ☐ Yes ☐ No ☐ N/A ☐
		An HgA1C value was on the patient's chart from Pre-Surgical Testing or Surgeon's office?	Yes ☐ No ☐
		Body Mass Index (BMI): 1 BMI >40? If yes, a wound vacuum dressing/drainage system was considered and available?	BMI:____________ Yes ☐ No ☐ N/A ☐
	Completed by:		(Print Name)
Operating Room (OR)	Circulating RN	Temperature upon arrival to the operating room?	Temperature:________
		Was the patient's abdomen prepped with CHG containing preparation when applicable?	Yes ☐ No ☐ NA ☐
		What was used for the vaginal preparation? ☐ Providone Iodine ☐ Irrisept ☐ 4% CHG	Yes ☐ No ☐ NA ☐
	Completed by:		(Print Name)
	Anesthesiologist	Was initial antibiotic prophylaxis selection and dosing given?	Yes ☐ No ☐
		Core temperature was checked every 30 minutes and maintained ≥36°C?	Yes ☐ No ☐
		If temperature < 36°C action is taken?	Yes ☐ No ☐ NA ☐
		What warming method(s) were used: ☐ Forced Air ☐ Fluid Warmer ☐ Other:____________	
		Glucose level was maintained < 200 mg/dL?	Yes ☐ No ☐
		When applicable was re-dosing of antibiotics given within the appropriate time?	Yes ☐ No ☐ NA ☐
		Did the patient receive hyper oxygenation: FIO2 > 80% in absence of contraindications?	Yes ☐ No ☐
		Was there an infection Present At the Time Of Surgery (PATOS)	Yes ☐ No ☐
		Assigned ASA: 1 2 3 4 5 The appropriate ASA Score was assigned?	Yes ☐ No ☐
	Completed by:		(Print Name)
	Circulating RN	Time Out: The wound was classified as: ☐ Clean (I) ☐ Clean/Contaminated (II) ☐ Contaminated (III) ☐ Dirty (IV)	
		Was a wound protector used?	Yes ☐ No ☐
		Was a sterile tray used at the time of closure?	Yes ☐ No ☐ NA ☐
		If wound class III or IV, were gowns and gloves changed before closing?	Yes ☐ No ☐
	Completed by:		(Print Name)
Post Anesthesia Care Unit	PACU RN or Post-Procedure RN	1. What was the patient's temperature on arrival to the PACU? (Goal 36°C - 38°C) 2. If temperature < 36°C, indicate action taken: ☐ Bair Hugger ☐ Other	Yes ☐ No ☐ Yes ☐ No ☐ NA ☐
		Patient's blood glucose maintained? (Goal < 200 mg/dL for applicable patients)	Yes ☐ No ☐
	Completed by:		(Print Name)

3.3 Antibiotic prophylaxis

The degree of contamination at the time of surgery is classified using the National Healthcare Safety Network (NHSN) wound class. Hysterectomy is a clean-contaminated procedure and as a result, is unavoidably associated with a relatively higher risk of infection as the procedure breaches the genital tract. Common sites of infection after hysterectomy include the abdominal wall, the vaginal cuff, bladder, and pelvic floor. Related complications include pelvic abscess or infected hematoma and sepsis. A patient's individual susceptibility to infection depends on a variety of factors including bacterial virulence, extent of surgery-related tissue trauma and fluid collection, the effectiveness of the patient's immune system, age, nutritional status, presence of diabetes, smoking, coexistent infection or colonization with microorganisms. Perhaps the most important factors in SSI prevention in hysterectomy are timely administration of appropriate preoperative antibiotics and meticulous surgical technique. Use of β-lactam alternatives in patients who do not report an anaphylactic reaction can lead to increased antimicrobial resistance. In fact, a retrospective cohort study involving over 21,000 women undergoing hysterectomy demonstrated that the use of standard β-lactam antibiotics had a lower risk of SSI compared to those who received an alternative regimen [23]. Thus, we advise judicious use of β-lactam alternatives for patients with a history of IgE-mediated penicillin hypersensitivity. The most common organisms isolated from vaginal cuff infections are anaerobes. In a large retrospective cohort study with over 18,000 patients undergoing hysterectomy of any type, those receiving cefazolin or a second-generation cephalosporin have more than double the SSI risk compared with those receiving combined treatment with cefazolin and metronidazole [25]. This is likely related to enhanced anaerobic coverage with the addition of metronidazole. We recommend that all patients undergoing hysterectomy receive metronidazole in addition to the standard intraoperative antibiotics.

3.4 Skin and vaginal preparation

The CDC also advises that the entire body be cleansed with either soap or antiseptic the night prior to the procedure. Intraoperatively, alcohol-based chlorhexidine is more effective for skin preparation when compared to iodine solutions [30, 31]. With regards to vaginal preparation, either povidone-iodine or chlorhexidine gluconate (4%) with a low concentration of isopropyl alcohol is acceptable, as both significantly reduce rates of postoperative infectious morbidity [32].

3.5 Post-hysterectomy care and precautions

In general, our practice will have patients return for short-term postoperative evaluation within 2 weeks following their hysterectomy. Patients are counseled to maintain pelvic rest for a minimum of 8 weeks. Postoperative blood and other secretions from the vaginal cuff may raise the vaginal pH and as a result, increase the risk of bacterial vaginosis. Many patients with vaginal cuff infections present more than 2 weeks following hysterectomy, which suggests a late ascending spread of vaginal microorganisms. As a result, our patients return for a second postoperative appointment and vaginal cuff check approximately 4–6 weeks after their hysterectomy.

4. Treatment

Gynecological surgical site infections are polymicrobial with a mix of both anaerobic and aerobic infections. Common pathogens contain gram-negative bacilli, enterococci, streptococci, and anaerobes—that is, *Staphylococcus aureus*, coagulase-negative staphylococci, and Streptococcus and Enterococcus species. When SSI is suspected, the wound should be thoroughly inspected. Surgical site infections are characterized as superficial, deep incisional, or organ/space. Involvement of the fascia and/or muscle with infection is the hallmark of a deep incisional SSI, whereas patients with organ/space SSI typically present with generalized malaise, fever, and pain. It becomes important to note that early recognition of necrotizing soft tissue infection is crucial. These infections can manifest rapidly after surgery with Group A streptococcus and clostridia as the primary pathogens.

Wound exploration and debridement are pillars in the management of superficial and deep-incisional SSIs. This includes not only opening the wound, debridement of necrotic and devitalized tissue, but also involves the culture of the wound to allow for speciation of potential pathogens to assist in antibiotic therapy.

The mortality and morbidity of organ/space SSI tend to be higher than superficial or deep SSI. The primary objective in management is to achieve source control. Computed tomography and ultrasound are employed to guide placement of closed suction percutaneous drains into abscess collections when feasible. The initial approach in treatment of post-hysterectomy pelvic abscess depends on three factors: (1) hemodynamic stability, (2) abscess size, and (3) abscess location. Hemodynamically unstable patients require prompt surgical intervention and intensive care monitoring.

Patients who are hemodynamically stable with a post-hysterectomy pelvic abscess should be treated empirically with parenteral broad-spectrum antibiotics. Initial antimicrobial regimens can be tailored to subsequent culture and sensitivity results. If the patient does not respond within 48–72 hours, percutaneous drainage or infectious disease consultation may be warranted. An argument can be made for earlier percutaneous drainage. In fact, a systematic review comparing the success rates of 3 modalities of minimally invasive management of tubo-ovarian abscesses—laparoscopy, ultrasound-guided drainage and computed tomography-guided drainage—reported that better outcomes were achieved by the minimally invasive approach when compared with conservative management. Of these techniques, image-guided drainage provided the highest success rates, fewest complications, and shortest hospital stay compared to laparoscopy [33].

Treatment failure is defined as persistent fever, leukocytosis, pain or lack of abscess resolution. Risk factors include residual fluid collection after drainage and increasing patient age. Surgical management is recommended at this time.

5. Summary

The most common reason for unplanned readmission after surgery is surgical site infection. SSIs are associated with increased morbidity, mortality, transfer to an intensive care setting, prolonged hospitalization, hospital readmission, and increased healthcare costs. In addition, the development of SSI negatively impacts patient experience.

The majority of postoperative issues can be anticipated and prevented preoperatively. Systematically addressing these issues at the preoperative evaluation may result in greater patient satisfaction and fewer complications. Thus, prevention of SSI after hysterectomy begins with a calculation of perioperative risk followed by addressing those risk factors prior to the procedure. Intraoperative measures aimed at SSI prevention include the implementation of evidence-based SSI prevention bundles, proper administration of intraoperative antibiotic prophylaxis, and proper skin/vaginal preparation. Postoperatively, hysterectomy patients should be followed closely.

Acknowledgements

Thanks to the faculty, residents, fellows, and medical students of the Zucker School of Medicine.

DOI: http://dx.doi.org/10.5772/intechopen.101492

Author details

Catherine W. Chan and Michael L. Nimaroff*
Northwell Health/Zucker School of Medicine, NY, USA

*Address all correspondence to: mnimaroff@northwell.edu

References

[1] Merrill RM. Hysterectomy surveillance in the United States, 1997 through 2005. Medical Science Monitor. 2008;**14**(1):CR24-CR31

[2] Wallace SK, Fazzari MJ, Chen H, Cliby WA, Chalas E. Outcomes and postoperative complications after hysterectomies performed for benign compared with malignant indications. Obstetrics and Gynecology. 2016;**128**(3): 467-475

[3] Wright JD, Herzog TJ, Tsui J, Ananth CV, Lewin SN, Lu Y-S, et al. Nationwide trends in the performance of inpatient hysterectomy in the United States. Obstetrics and Gynecology. 2013;**122**(2 Pt 1):233-241

[4] Edwards JR, Peterson KD, Andrus ML, Dudeck MA, Pollock DA, Horan TC. National healthcare safety network (NHSN) report, data summary for 2006 through 2007, issued November 2008. American Journal of Infection Control. 2008;**36**(9):609-626

[5] Mahdi H, Goodrich S, Lockhart D, DeBernardo R, Moslemi-Kebria M. Predictors of surgical site infection in women undergoing hysterectomy for benign gynecologic disease: A multicenter analysis using the national surgical quality improvement program data. Journal of Minimally Invasive Gynecology. 2014;**21**(5):901-909

[6] Uppal S, Harris J, Al-Niaimi A, Swenson CW, Pearlman MD, Reynolds RK, et al. Prophylactic antibiotic choice and risk of surgical site infection after hysterectomy. Obstetrics and Gynecology. 2016;**127**(2):321-329

[7] Gandaglia G, Ghani KR, Sood A, Meyers JR, Sammon JD, Schmid M, et al. Effect of minimally invasive surgery on the risk for surgical site infections: Results from the national surgical quality improvement program (NSQIP) database. JAMA Surgery. 2014; **149**(10):1039-1044

[8] Andiman SE, Xu X, Boyce JM, Ludwig EM, Rillstone HRW, Desai VB, et al. Decreased surgical site infection rate in hysterectomy: Effect of a gynecology-specific bundle. Obstetrics and Gynecology. 2018;**131**(6): 991-999

[9] Steinberg JP, Braun BI, Hellinger WC, Kusek L, Bozikis MR, Bush AJ, et al. Timing of antimicrobial prophylaxis and the risk of surgical site infections: Results from the trial to reduce antimicrobial prophylaxis errors. Annals of Surgery. 2009;**250**(1):10-16

[10] Roy S, Patkar A, Daskiran M, Levine R, Hinoul P, Nigam S. Clinical and economic burden of surgical site infection in hysterectomy. Surgical Infections. 2014;**15**(3):266-273

[11] Committee opinion no. 701 summary: Choosing the route of hysterectomy for benign disease. Obstetrics and Gynecology. 2017;**129**(6): 1149-1150

[12] Lake AG, McPencow AM, Dick-Biascoechea MA, Martin DK, Erekson EA. Surgical site infection after hysterectomy. American Journal of Obstetrics and Gynecology. 2013;**209**(5):490.e1-490.e9

[13] Aarts JWM, Nieboer TE, Johnson N, Tavender E, Garry R, Mol BWJ, et al. Surgical approach to hysterectomy for benign gynaecological disease. Cochrane Database of Systematic Reviews. 2015;**8**:CD003677

[14] Brown O, Geynisman-Tan J, Gillingham A, Collins S, Lewicky-Gaupp C, Kenton K, et al. Minimizing risks in minimally invasive surgery: Rates of surgical site infection across subtypes of laparoscopic hysterectomy.

Journal of Minimally Invasive Gynecology. 2020;**27**(6):1370-1376.e1

[15] Moulton L, Jernigan AM, Carr C, Freeman L, Escobar PF, Michener CM. Single-port laparoscopy in gynecologic oncology: Seven years of experience at a single institution. American Journal of Obstetrics and Gynecology. 2017;**217**(5): 610.e1-610.e8

[16] Nimaroff ML, Crihfield E. Single port laparoscopic assisted hysterectomy. In: Single Port Gynecologic Laparoscopic and Robotic-Assisted Surgery. IntechOpen; 2021

[17] Sherer DM, Schwartz BM, Abulafia O. Management of pelvic abscess during pregnancy: A case and review of the literature. Obstetrical & Gynecological Survey. 1999;**54**(10): 655-662

[18] Matsunaga Y, Fukushima K, Nozaki M, Nakanami N, Kawano Y, Shigematsu T, et al. A case of pregnancy complicated by the development of a tubo-ovarian abscess following in vitro fertilization and embryo transfer. American Journal of Perinatology. 2003;**20**(6):277-282

[19] Al-Kuran O, Beitawi S, Al-Mehaisen L. Pelvic abscess complicating an in vitro fertilization pregnancy and review of the literature. Journal of Assisted Reproduction and Genetics. 2008;**25**(7):341-343

[20] Patounakis G, Krauss K, Nicholas SS, Baxter JK, Rosenblum NG, Berghella V. Development of pelvic abscess during pregnancy following transvaginal oocyte retrieval and in vitro fertilization. European Journal of Obstetrics, Gynecology, and Reproductive Biology. 2012;**164**(1):116-117

[21] Martin ET, Kaye KS, Knott C, Nguyen H, Santarossa M, Evans R, et al. Diabetes and risk of surgical site infection: A systemic review and meta-analysis. Infection Control and Hospital Epidemiology. 2016;**37**(1):88-99

[22] Perioperative pathways: Enhanced recovery after surgery: ACOG committee opinion no. 750. Obstetrics and Gynecology. 2018;**132**:e120-e130

[23] Soper DE. Gynecologic sequelae of bacterial vaginosis. International Journal of Gynaecology and Obstetrics. 1999;**67**(Suppl. 1):S25-S28

[24] Stone R, Carey E, Fader AN, Fitzgerald J, Hammons L, Nensi A, et al. Enhanced recovery and surgical optimization protocol for minimally invasive gynecologic surgery: An AAGL white paper. Journal of Minimally Invasive Gynecology. 2021;**28**(2): 179-203

[25] Till SR, Morgan DM, Bazzi AA, Pearlman MD, Abdelsattar Z, Campbell DA, et al. Reducing surgical site infections after hysterectomy: Metronidazole plus cefazolin compared with cephalosporin alone. American Journal of Obstetrics and Gynecology. 2017;**217**(2):187.e1-187.e11

[26] Ma N, Cameron A, Tivey D, Grae N, Roberts S, Morris A. Systematic review of a patient care bundle in reducing staphylococcal infections in cardiac and orthopaedic surgery. ANZ Journal of Surgery. 2017;**87**(4):239-246

[27] Vij SC, Kartha G, Krishnamurthi V, Ponziano M, Goldman HB. Simple operating room bundle reduces superficial surgical site infections after major urologic surgery. Urology. 2018;**112**:66-68

[28] Carter EB, Temming LA, Fowler S, Eppes C, Gross G, Srinivas SK, et al. Evidence-based bundles and cesarean delivery surgical site infections: A systematic review and meta-analysis. Obstetrics and Gynecology. 2017;**130**(4): 735-746

[29] Pellegrini JE, Toledo P, Soper DE, Bradford WC, Cruz DA, Levy BS, et al. Consensus bundle on prevention of surgical site infections after major gynecologic surgery. Obstetrics and Gynecology. 2017;**129**(1):50-61

[30] Berríos-Torres SI, Umscheid CA, Bratzler DW, Leas B, Stone EC, Kelz RR, et al. Centers for disease control and prevention guideline for the prevention of surgical site infection, 2017. JAMA Surgery. 2017;**152**(8):784-791

[31] Prevention of infection after gynecologic procedures: ACOG practice bulletin summary, number 195. Obstetrics and Gynecology. 2018;**131**(6): 1177-1179

[32] Skeith AE, Morgan DM, Schmidt PC. Vaginal preparation with povidone-iodine or chlorhexidine before hysterectomy: A propensity score matched analysis. American Journal of Obstetrics and Gynecology. 2021 Nov 1;**225**(5):560.e1560.e9. DOI: 10.1016/j.ajog.2021.08.035

[33] Goje O, Markwei M, Kollikonda S, Chavan M, Soper DE. Outcomes of minimally invasive management of tubo-ovarian abscess: A systematic review. Journal of Minimally Invasive Gynecology. 2021;**28**(3):556-564

Chapter 7

Cases of Postpartum Hemorrhage and Hysterectomy in Thailand's Northern and Northeastern Provincial Hospitals

Thawalsak Ratanasiri, Natakorn I. Tuporn, Somnuk Apiwantanagul, Thitima Nutrawong, Thawalrat Ratanasiri and Amornrat Ratanasiri

Abstract

PPH is a major cause of maternal death. Hysterectomy is safe to treat uncontrollable PPH. However, it may not be the best option for women who want to have children. The risk score tool to detect PPH earlier is needed in low-resource cities such as Chiang Rai and Sakon Nakhon province. This study aims to perform a risk score tool to prevent PPH in the northern and northeastern hospitals in Thailand; using mixed methods, identify risk factors for PPH from 20 articles globally and in Thailand using Med Calc, and develop the tool for prediction of PPH; and tool testing and a one-year follow-up on PPH-related hysterectomy cases. Results showed that this risk score tool can detect PPH earlier, reducing the number of PPH and hysterectomy cases. This risk score tool needs to be implemented in the same situations as hospitals to save pregnant women's lives.

Keywords: PPH reduction, hysterectomy, Chiang Rai regional hospital, and Sakon Nakhon hospital

1. Introduction

Hemorrhage is the cause of 12.0–18.0% of deaths during pregnancy [1–3]. Severe postpartum hemorrhage (PPH) is a major cause of maternal mortality and morbidity [4, 5] and is increasing in incidence worldwide [6, 7], especially in low resource countries [8]. Emergency hysterectomy is increasingly performed to treat uncontrollable PPH [1–3]. It was performed at the time of, or within 24 h of, a vaginal or abdominal delivery for the treatment of hemorrhage that was unresponsive to unservative approaches [9]. Variability in the incidence of PPH-related hysterectomy is different in various countries and even among institutions [9–13].

According to recent reports, 0.20–5.09 of every 1000 postnatal women across the globe have undergone an emergency hysterectomy [14]. Hysterectomy is considered to be a safe, low-risk surgery. It is, by nature, unplanned and performed expeditiously in the case of severe PPH. It may not be the best option for all women, especially those

IntechOpen

who still want to have children. Some people may have an adverse reaction to the anesthetic, heavy bleeding, and infection around the incision site [15].

The guidelines of the World Health Organization (WHO) aim to prevent and manage PPH by active management of the third stage of labor (AMTSL) [16]. Thai government policy to prevent PPH in 2013 was involved in the project—Every Woman Every Child (EWEC) to decrease maternal mortality and child mortality by 16 million cases in 2015 [17, 18]. However, the incidence of PPH was increased from 2.30 to 2.65% from 2009 to 2015 [19]. In low-resource city with various ethnic groups, surrounded by mountains and forests as in Chiang Rai province and Sakon Nakhon province [20, 21]. The incidence of PPH is increasing in Chiang Rai from 1.12 to 2.07%, but maternal death from PPH decreased from 3.05 to 1.23% during 2012-2015 [20]. In the fiscal year 2014–2015, PPH-related hysterectomy decreased in number from 2 cases to 1 case [20]. In Sakon Nakhon, during 2015–2018 the incidence of PPH is about 1.13–1.39%. The maternal deaths were decreased from 33.83 to 27.84 per 100,000 infant live births. However, it was higher than the standard criterion of 17.0 per 100,000 infant live births [21].

A tool developed from significantly high-risk factors [22–24] associated with PPH was performed in western societies and Thailand [25–29]. These tools can detect PPH earlier and can reduce the number of maternal deaths and PPH-related hysterectomies in Thailand [20, 21].

This study aimed to synthesize knowledge about the early management of PPH, summarize the appropriate risk score tool for the prediction of PPH, and reduce the number of maternal deaths and PPH-related hysterectomy cases in two lower resource cities in the north and northeast of Thailand.

2. Objectives

The objective of this study was to synthesize knowledge about the early management of PPH and an appropriate risk score tool to reduce PPH-related hysterectomy cases in two lower resource cities in the north and northeast of Thailand.

3. Methodologies

The study reviewed the results of the author's research in four steps as follows:

Step 1: Using meta-analysis, we reviewed the risk factors for PPH during vaginal deliveries in 20 articles published in Thailand and around the world between 2005 and 2017.

Step 2: Reviewed the research results of the risk scoring system for the prediction of postpartum blood loss over 300 mL at Chiang Rai Regional Hospital, Thailand.

Step 3: Reviewed the research results of an appropriate risk score tool for the prediction of PPH at Sakon Nakhon Hospital, Thailand.

Step 4: During the years 2019–2020, the number of maternal deaths and PPH-related hysterectomies at Chiang Rai Regional Hospital and Sakon Nakhon province were reported.

The research review was approved by the Ethics Committee for Human Research at Khon Kaen University, Thailand [HE 601234, HE 611093], the Chiang Rai Regional Hospital Ethics Committee on July 21st, 2017, and the Ethics committee of Sakon Nakhon Hospital (SKHREC 422562). Most of the research was based on secondary data. Those who volunteered had signed a consent form.

DOI: http://dx.doi.org/10.5772/intechopen.102948

4. Results

There are four steps to this research result as follows:

In Step 1, reviewed research results of risk factors for PPH via vaginal deliveries: systematic review and meta-analysis (**Table 1**) [29].

Risk factors	Subgroup	Statistical procedures		
		Heterogeneity Test I^2	Estimate size (fixed effect)	
			OR (95% CI)	*P*-value
I. Eight of high-risk factors (odds ratio > 2.0)				
1. Antepartum hemoglobin level	>10 g/dL	95.71	4.80 (4.00–5.76)	<0.001
2. Coagulopathy		35.18	11.96 (2.64–54.10)	0.004
3. History of prior pregnancy and delivery	Prior PPH	40.89	4.01 (2.32–6.93)	<0.001
4. Complication of current pregnancy, 1st stage of labor, received procedure of 1st stage of labor	Fibroid	89.97	0.73 (0.70–0.75)	<0.001
5. Complication of current pregnancy, 1st stage of labor, received procedure of 1st stage of labor	Multiple pregnancy	51.23	2.69 (2.32–3.11)	<0.001
6. Complication of current pregnancy, 1st stage of labor, received procedure of 1st stage of labor	Gestational hypertensive disorder	69.13	2.07 (1.72–2.50)	<0.001
7. Placenta factors	Placenta previa	28.44	5.01 (3.61–6.97)	<0.001
8. Placenta Factors	Placenta accrete	0.00	3.55 (1.84–6.86)	<0.001
II. Six moderate risk factors (odds ratio > 1.5–2.0)				
1. Obstetric factors parity	Nulliparous	72.62	1.93 (1.53–2.43)	<0.001
2. Gestational age (large gestational age)	>40 weeks	47.19	1.35 (1.28–1.42)	<0.001
3. Placenta factors	Placenta abruption	39.13	1.70 (1.06–2.73)	0.029
4. Complication of current pregnancy, 1st stage of labor, received procedure of 1st stage of labor	Chorioamnionitis	0.00	1.85 (1.45–2.98)	0.012
5. Complication of current pregnancy, 1st stage of labor, received procedure of 1st stage of labor	Induction of labor	69.33	1.77 (1.57–2.00)	<0.001
6. Complication of current pregnancy, 1st stage of labor, received procedure of 1st stage of labor	Augmentation of Labor	69.66	1.57 (1.35–5.87)	<0.001
III. Seven of low-risk factors (odds ratio > 1.0–1.5)				
1. Individual factors maternal age	<20 years old	31.40	1.36 (1.26–1.46)	<0.001

Risk factors	Subgroup	Statistical procedures		
		Heterogeneity Test I^2	Estimate size (fixed effect)	
			OR (95% CI)	*P*-value
2. Individual factors maternal age	>35 years old	17.37	1.32 (1.29–1.35)	<0.001
3. 1 Body mass index (BMI) level	<30 kg/m^2	0.00	1.17 (1.05–1.31)	0.050
3. 2 Body mass index (BMI) level	>30 kg/m^2	0.00	1.18 (1.01–1.38)	0.027
4. Obstetric Factors parity	Primiparous	97.64	1.29 (1.18–1.41)	<0.001
5. Gestational age	>42 weeks	47.19	1.35 (1.28–1.42)	<0.001
6. Complication of current pregnancy, 1st stage of labor, received procedure of 1st stage of labor	Gestational diabetes mellitus	0.00	1.35 (1.22–1.45)	<0.001
7. Complication of current pregnancy and 1st stage of labor receive procedure	Received analgesic drugs	10.03	1.38 (1.27–1.49)	<0.001

Source: approved by I-Tuporn, et al. [29].

Table 1.
Med calc version 18.6 was used to analyze risk factors for PPH during vaginal deliveries.

Form for Recording Risk Scores to predict Postpartum Hemorrhage (PPH)

Predictors	Score	Pt Score	Criteria
1.Age > 35 years old	3		[ ] Low risk score < 4 (EBL < 300 ml.)
2.Gestational age >40 weeks	2		
3.Nulliparous	2		
4.Curettage in prior pregnancy	4		[ ] High risk score ≥ 4 (EBL > 300 ml.)
5.Gestational hypertensive disorder	7		
6.Hemoglobin < 10 gram per deciliters	8		
7.Fundal height > 38 centimeters	2		
8.Having received pethidine for pain relief in the 1st stage of labor	2		
Total score	30		

Type of delivery [ ] ND [ ] V/E [ ] F/E [ ] BA [ ] VBAC

Total blood loss from collector bag _______ ml.

Others 1. Medication to prevent or treat PPH...

2. Surgery for the safety of pregnant women from uncontrollable PPH (Hysterectomy for PPH)

Figure 1.
Form for recording risk scores to predict postpartum hemorrhage (PPH) of blood loss over 300 ml after vaginal delivery. Source: approved by I-Tuporn, et al. [31].

Level of blood loss	ROC curve	Sensitivity (%)	Specificity (%)	Accuracy (%)	Positive predictive value (%)	Negative predictive value (%)	95% CI	P-Value
>250 ml	0.627	57.33	61.95	59.84	58.01	61.48	0.592–0.662	<0.001
>275 ml	0.608	15.69	92.92	56.04	66.96	54.66	0.554–0.662	<0.001
>300 ml	0.606	15.48	92.92	55.94	66.66	54.60	0.552–0.661	<0.001
>500 ml	0.653	5.02	98.66	53.94	77.41	53.19	0.563–0.744	0.004

Source: Approved by Nutravong et al. [35], on An Appropriate Assessment of PPH by using a Risk Score Tool for prediction at Sakon Nakhon, Hospital, Thailand oral presentation in the International Webinar on Primary Healthcare and Medicare held during November 08–09, 2021/Vienna Austria.

Table 2.
Review of risk score at the different levels of blood loss from 250 ml. to 500 ml. in 1001 cases who underwent vaginal delivery at Sakhon Nakhon hospital, Thailand, during June 2018 to December 2019.

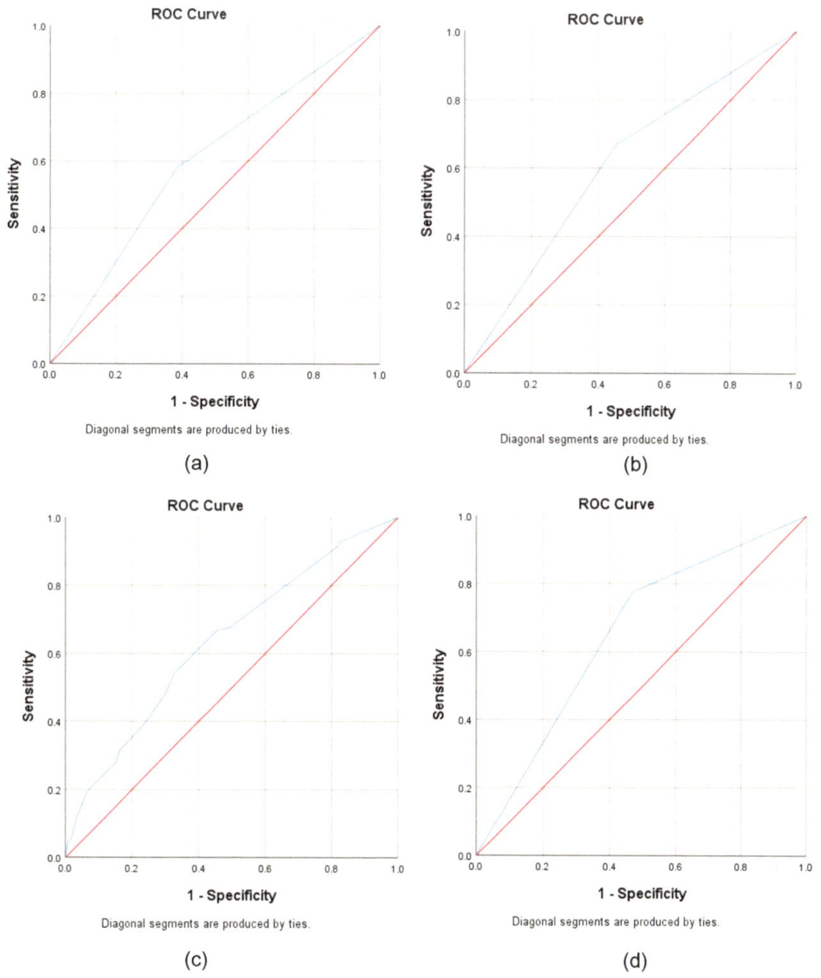

Figure 2.
The ROC curve's performance at different levels of blood loss at over (a) 250 mL, (b) 275 mL, (c) 300 mL, and (d) 500 mL of a risk score for PPH prediction from 1001 cases after delivery at Sakon Nakhon hospital, Thailand from July 2018 to December 2019.

Setting	Pregnancy Problems	Fiscal years											
		2009	2010	2011	2012	2013	2014	2015	2016	2017	2018	2019	2020
Thailand*	Incidence of PPH	2.30%	2.37%	2.44%	2.40%	2.39%	2.54%	2.65%	NA	NA	NA	NA	NA
Chiang Rai** Province	Incidence of PPH	NA	NA	NA	1.12%	1.15%	1.34%	2.07%	NA	NA	NA	NA	NA
	PPH related Hysterectomy	NA	NA	NA	NA	NA	2	1 case	NA	NA	NA	NA	NA
	Maternal death/100,000 infant live birth	NA	NA	NA	3.05	4.58	1.82	1.23	NA	NA	NA	NA	NA
Chiang Rai** Regional Hospital	Incidence of PPH	NA	NA	NA	NA	9.0%	1.98%	2.64%	2.58%	2.61%	3.85%	4.61%	3.81%
	PPH related Hysterectomy	NA	NA	NA	NA	1 case	NA	NA	NA	NA	NA	NA	NA
	Maternal death/ 100,000 infant live birth	NA	NA	NA	NA	NA	36.14	18.09	NA	NA	17.45	36.60	37.36
Sakon Nakhon*** Province	Incidence of PPH	NA	NA	NA	NA	NA	NA	1.13%	0.93%	1.00%	1.39%	1.10%	NA
	PPH related Hysterectomy	NA	NA	NA	NA	NA	NA	NA	NA	NA	NA	NA	NA
	Maternal death/100,000 infant live birth	NA	NA	NA	NA	NA	NA	33.83	17.68	26.88	27.84	15.12	NA

**Medical Department, Ministry of Public Health document 2013 [17].*
***Ajalapung, 2015 [20].*
****Statistic Report for NE Thailand, 2019 [21].*
Remarks: The standard Criterion of maternal deaths was 17 per 100,000 infant live birth.

Table 3.
Statistics on PPH, PPH-related hysterectomy, and maternal deaths were collected in Thailand's Chiang Rai Province. Chiang Rai regional hospital, Sakon Nakhon Province.

This study was analyzed and identified risk factors for PPH via vaginal deliveries from 20 articles from 2005 to 2017 in Thailand and globally, using MedCalc version 18.2.1 and version 18.6 [30].

The results showed that 21 factors, including eight high-risk factors for PPH (odds ratio > 2.0) include antepartum hemoglobin ≤10 g/dL, coagulopathy, prior PPH, fibroid, placenta previa, placenta accrete, multiple pregnancy, and gestational hypertensive disorder. Six moderate risk factors for PPH (odds ratio > 1.5–2.0) include nulliparous status, large gestational age, placenta abruption, chorioamnionitis, induction, and augmentation of labor. Seven low-risk factors for PPH (odds ratio > 1.0–1.5) include maternal age < 20 years old and ≥ 35 years old, BMI level, primiparous, gestational age ≥ 42 weeks, gestational diabetes mellitus, and having received analgesic drugs.

In Step 2, Chiang Rai Regional Hospital reviewed the research findings of a risk scoring system for predicting postpartum blood loss greater than 300 mL (**Figure 1**) [31].

The results showed that the eight predictors of I-Tuporn et al. [31] (**Figure 1**) from the cause of PPH (4 T's and 7 steps of the clinical prediction model of Steyerberg) [32, 33] and by comparison with the standard monogram of Biguzzi [34], Sittipan [28], and Suta [27] could predict postpartum blood loss over 300 ml at Chiang Rai Regional Hospital with a sensitivity of 80.7%, a specificity of 60.8%, and the ROC curve equal to 0.71 at the optional cut-off score of four marks or above (see **Figure 1**) [31].

In Step 3, we reviewed research results for an appropriate assessment of PPH by. using a risk score tool for prediction at Sakon Nakhon Hospital, Thailand (**Table 2**) [35].

It found that the eight predictors of I-Tuporn et al. [31] (**Figure 1**) can be used to predict early PPH in Sakon Nakhon Hospital since blood loss is 250 ml and over with a sensitivity of 57.33%, a specificity of 61.95%, and a ROC curve equal to 0.62 (**Table 2** and **Figure 2**).

In Step 4, We reported the number of maternal deaths and PPH-related hysterectomy at Chiang Rai Regional Hospital and Sakon Nakhon province during 2019–2020.

The results of one-year follow-up showed the incidence of Chiang Rai Regional Hospital.

The number of cases of PPH-related hysterectomy decreased from 4.61% to 3.81% from 2019 to 2020 report of. It had no cases of PPH-related hysterectomy but had reported no maternal death per 100,000 infant live births, 36.60 and 37.36 respectively.

In Sakon Nakhon province, the incidence of PPH decreased from 1.39 to 1.10%, but there was no report of PPH-related hysterectomy. The maternal death rate decreased from 27.84 to 15.12 per 100,000 live births, from 2018 to 2019 (**Table 3**).

5. Discussions

The postpartum hemorrhage (PPH) in I-Tuporn et al. [31] study, which was conducted in the Chiang Rai Regional Hospital in 2017, was 2.61%. It was lower than the study in Chonburi Hospital (4.95%) [28] and Maharat Nakorn Ratchasima Hospital (6.67%) [26], but it was related to the report of Bhumibol Adulyadej Hospital (1.98%) [25] and the report of Calvert et al. [36] that presented Asia's regional PPH rate of 1.90% [36].

Emergency hysterectomy for the treatment of severe hemorrhage from vaginal delivery was not reported widely in Chiang Rai Regional Hospital or Sakon Nakhon province. It was presented only some years ago and reported only a few cases. However, the maternal death rate in Sakon Nakhon province from 2015 to 2018 was higher than the standard criterion of 17 per 100,000 infant live births. It was decreased in the year 2019 to 15.12 per 100,000 infant live births after this hospital used a risk score tool with 8 predictors by I-Tuporn et al. [31] to detect earlier PPH and early treatment as blood loss over 250 mL from the collector bag.

The risk score tool for the prediction of PPH in Thailand had five studies [25–29]. They were developed in different settings. They had some similar risk factors for the detection of PPH. The study of I-Tuporn et al. [31] developed the risk score tool with 8 predictors, covering the cause of PPH (4 T's and 7 steps of the clinical prediction model of Steyerberg [32, 33] and by comparison with the standard monogram of Biguzzi [34], Sittipan [28], and Suta et al. [27]) I-Tuporn et al. [31] risk score tool could be used in low-resource cities with various ethnic groups, as in Chiang Rai and Sakon Nakhon province, which are in the north and northeast of Thailand, respectively.

The results of the Chiang Rai and Sakon Nakhon provinces study after 1 year of follow-up showed that the maternal death rate in Sakon Nakhon province had decreased to normal criterion, and there were no reports of PPH-related hysterectomy cases in these two provinces.

6. Conclusions

In conclusion, the problems of PPH concerned the Thai government. Many projects were carried out in accordance with World Health Organization's (WHO) [16] guidelines to reduce PPH, PPH-related hysterectomy, and maternal death.

Due to some settings in Thailand, the government's policy is not suitable for some women because of their low resources and distance from the cities. Some of the settings are surrounded by mountains and forests, and it is very hard to refer a pregnant woman with PPH to the provincial hospital. Most of them belong to different ethnic groups and cannot communicate with other people. Therefore, some of them die before seeing a doctor.

There should be a policy of early detection of PPH in those lower resource settings by using an appropriate risk score tool to predict the PPH risk for a pregnant woman's life.

Acknowledgements

The authors would like to thank all of the respondents for their valuable contributions to this study and extend their special gratitude to the Department of Obstetrics and Gynecology in Chiang Rai Regional Hospital and Sakon Nakhon Hospital for the data support, and the Thai Society of Maternal and Fetal Medicine for funding support.

Conflict of interest

All authors declare that they have no conflicts of interest.

Author details

Thawalsak Ratanasiri[1], Natakorn I. Tuporn[2], Somnuk Apiwantanagul[3], Thitima Nutrawong[4], Thawalrat Ratanasiri[4] and Amornrat Ratanasiri[5]*

1 Khon Kaen Hospital, Khon Kaen, Thailand

2 Chiang Rai College, Chiang Rai, Thailand

3 Sakon Nakhon Hospital, Sakon Nakhon, Thailand

4 Faculty of Medicine, Khon Kaen University, Khon Kaen, Thailand

5 Faculty of Medicine, Department of Community Medicine, Khon Kaen University, Khon Kaen, Thailand

*Address all correspondence to: amorat@kku.ac.th

References

[1] Clark SL, Belfort MA, Dildy GA, Herbst MA, Meyers JA, Hankins GD. Maternal death in the 21st Century, causes, prevention, and relationship to cesarean delivery. American Journal of Obstetrics and Gynecology. 2008;**199**: 36el-5. DOI: 10.1016/j.ajog.2008.03.007

[2] Creanga AA, Cl B, Syverson C, Seed K, Bruce FC, Callaghan WM. Pregnancy-related mortality in the United States, 2006-2010. Obstetrics and Gynecology. 2015;**125**:5-12. DOI: 10.1097/AOG.0000000000000564

[3] Saucedo M, Deneox-Tharnux C, Bouvier-Colle MH. Ten years of confidential inquiries into maternal deaths in France; 1998-2007. Obstetrics and Gynecology. 2013;**122**:752-760. DOI: 10.1097/AOG.0b013e31829fc38c

[4] Calleaghan WM, Kuklina EV, Berg CI. Trends in postpartum hemorrhage: United States, 1994-2006. American Journal of Obstetrics and Gynecology. 2010;**202**:353e1-6. DOI: 10.1016/j.ajog.2010.01.011

[5] Say L, Chou D, Gemmill A, Tunçalp Ö, Moller AB, Daniels J, et al. Global causes of maternal death: A WHO systematic analysis. The Lancet Global Health. 2014;**2**:e323-e333

[6] Mehrabadi A, Hutcheon JA, Lee L, Kramer MS, Liston RM, Joseph KS. Epidermiological investigation of a temporal increase in atonic program haemorrhage: A population-based retrospective cohort study. BJOG. 2013;**120**:853-862. DOI: 10.1111/1471-0528.12149

[7] Kramer MS, Berg C, Abenhaim H, Dahhou M, Rouleau J, Mehrabadi A, et al. Incidence, risk factors, and temporal trends in severe postpartum hemorrhage. American Journal of Obstetrics and Gynecology. 2013;**209**(449):e1-e7. DOI: 10.1016/j.ajog.2013.07.007

[8] Chersich M, Blaauw D, Dumbaugh M, Penn-Kekana L, Thwala S, Bijlmakers L, et al. Mapping of research on maternal health interventions in low- and middle-income countries: A review of 2292 publications between 2000 and 2012. Global Health. 2016;**12**:52. DOI: 10118681292-016-0189-1

[9] Zhang Y, Yan J, Han O, Yang T, Cai L, Fu Y, et al. Emergency obstetric hysterectomy for life-threatening postpartum hemorrhage: A 12-year review. Medicine (Baltimore). 2017;**96**:e8443. DOI: 10.1097/MD.0000000000008443

[10] Demirci O, Tugral AS, Yilmaz E, Tosun O, Demirci E, Eren YS. Emergency peripatum hysterectomy in a tertiary obstetric center: Nine years evaluation. American Journal of Obstetrics and Gynecology. 2011;**37**: 1054-1060. DOI: 10.1111/j.1447-0756.2010.01484. x

[11] Ozden S, Yildinin G, Baseran T, Turbuz B, Dayiciogle V. Analysis of 59 cases of emergent peripartum hysterectomies during a 13-years period. American Journal of Obstetrics and Gynecology. 2005;**271**:363-367. DOI: 10.1007/s00404-004-0647-5

[12] Kwee A, Bots ML, Visset GH, Bruinse HW. Emergency periparum hysterectomy: A prospective study in the Netherlands. European Journal of Obstetrics & Gynecology and Reproductive Biology. 2006;**124**:187-192. DOI: 10.1016/j.ejogrb.2005.06.012

[13] Baternam BT, Mihyre JM, Callingham WM, Kuklina E. Peripartum hysterectomy in the United States: nationwide 14-year experience. American Journal of Obstetrics and Gynecology. 2012;**206**(63):e1-e8. DOI: 10.1016/j.ajog.2011.07.030

[14] de la Cruz CZ, Thompson EL, O'Rourke K, Nembhard WN. Cesarean

section and the risk of emergency peripartum hysterectomy in high-income countries: A systematic review. Archives of Gynecology and Obstetrics. 2015;**292**:1201-1215. DOI: 10.1007/s00404-015-3790-2

[15] Kelbach J, Stang D. Hysterectomy. Available from: https://www.healthline.com/health/hysterectomy. [cited 2018 Jan 30]

[16] World Health Organization. WHO Recommendations for the Prevention and Treatment of Postpartum Hemorrhage. Geneva: World Health Organization; 2012

[17] Medical Department, Ministry of Public Health. Document of standard labor room in Ajulapong J. Problems solving for reduce maternal death from postpartum hemorrhage [presentation] Chiang Rai: Chiang Rai Prachanukroh Hospital; 2015.

[18] Saereeporncharenkul K. Development of quality labor room in Rajavithi hospital. Rajavithi Hospital News. 2015;**10**:1-15

[19] Limpanyalert P. How to Reduce Morbidity and Mortality of Postpartum Hemorrhage. Paper Presented at Workshop Proceeding of Community Practice for Patient Safety in Labor Rooms. Bangkok, Thailand: AFP; 2015

[20] Ajulapong J. Problems Solving for Reduce Maternal Death from Postpartum Hemorrhage [Presentation]. Chiang Rai, Chiang Rai Prachanukroh Hospital; 2015

[21] Statistical Report in Northeast of Thailand. Maternal death in 7 provinces, during 9 months (October, 2018 to June, 2019). [n.d]; Report A.1/CE, All Provincial Public Health Offices in Regional the eight. 2019 in Ratanasiri T, Apiwantanagul S, Ratanasiri A, Nutravong T. An appropriate assessment of postpartum hemorrhage by using a risk score tool for prediction at Sakon Nakhon Hospital, Thailand. Oral presentation in the International Webinar on Primary Healthcare and Medicare held during November 08-09, 2021/Vienna Austria

[22] Sheiner E, Sarid L, Levy A, Seidman DS, Hallak M. Obstetric risk factors and outcome of pregnancies complicated with early postpartum hemorrhage: A population-based study. The Journal of Maternal-Fetal & Neonatal Medicine. 2005;**18**:149-154. DOI: 10.1080/14767050500170088

[23] Briley A, Seed PT, Tydeman G, Ballard H, Waterstone M, Sandall J, et al. Reporting errors, incidence and risk factors for postpartum haemorrhage and progression to severe PPH: A prospective observational study. BJOG. 2014;**121**:876-888. DOI: 10.1111/1471-0528.12588

[24] Frass KA. Postpartum hemorrhage is related to the hemoglobin levels at labor: Observational study. Alexandria Journal of Medicine. 2015;**51**:333-337

[25] Rueangchainikhom W, Srisuwan S, Prommas S, Sarapak S. Risk factors for primary postpartum hemorrhage in Bhumibol Adulyadej hospital. Journal of the Medical Association of Thailand. 2009;**92**:1586-1590

[26] Sathapornteera P, Arj-Ong S. Factors associated with early postpartum hemorrhage of singleton pregnancy in Maharat Nakhon Ratchasima hospital. Thai Journal of Obstetrics and Gynaecology. 2012;**20**:21-28

[27] Suta J, Leungratsameerung S, Phaloprakarn C. A risk score for predicting postpartum hemorrhage in association with cesarean delivery. Thai Journal of Obstetrics and Gynaecology. 2015;**23**:3-11

[28] Sittiparn W, Siwadune T. Risk score for prediction of postpartum hemorrhages in normal labor at Chonburi

hospital. Journal of the Medical Association of Thailand. 2017;**100**:382-388

[29] I-Tuporn N, Ratanasiri A, Nutravong T, Boonprasert K, Napikul T. Risk factors for postpartum hemorrhage via vaginal deliveries: Systematic review and meta-analysis. Chiangrai Medical Journal. 2018;**10**:150-160

[30] Med Calc Version 18.2.1 (Free Trial Version 15 days). Available from: https://www.medcalc.org/download.php [cited 2018 Jan 30]

[31] I-Tuporn N, Ratanasiri A, Nutravong T, Boonprasert K, Napikul T, Risk scoring system for the prediction of postpartum blood loss over 300 mL at Chiang Rai regional hospital. The Siriraj Medical Journal. 2019;**72**(1):112-118

[32] Steyerberg EW. Clinical Prediction Models: A Practical Approach to Development, Validation, and Updating. New York: Springer; 2009

[33] Steyerberg EW, Vergouwe Y. Towards better clinical prediction models: Seven steps for development and an ABCD for validation. European Heart Journal. 2014;**35**:1925-1931

[34] Biguzzi E, Franchi F, Ambrogi E, Ibrahim B, Bucciarelli P, Acaia B, et al. Risk factors for postpartum hemorrhage in a cohort of 6,011 Italian women. Thrombosis Research. 2012;**129**:e1-e7

[35] Ratanasiri T, Apiwantanagul S, Ratanasiri A, Nutravong T. An appropriate assessment of postpartum hemorrhage by using a risk score tool for prediction at Sakon Nakhon Hospital, Thailand. In: Nutravong T, editor. Oral Presentation in the International Webinar on Primary Healthcare and Medicare Held During November 08-09, 2021/Vienna Austria. 2021

[36] Calvert C, Thomas SL, Ronsmans C, Wagner KS, Adler AJ, Filippi V. Identifying regional variation in the prevalence of postpartum hemorrhage: A systematic review and meta-analysis. PLoS One. 2012;**7**:e41114. DOI: 10.1371/journal.pone.0041114

Chapter 8

Management of Vaginal Vault Prolapse after Hysterectomy

Johnstone Shabaya Miheso

Abstract

Pelvic organ prolapse is described as the symptomatic downwards displacement of pelvic organs through the vagina. The incidence of pelvic organ prolapse is difficult to ascertain, but it is said to affect up to 50% of women worldwide over their lifetime. Majority are asymptomatic, but some will complain of a feeling of something coming down their vagina, discomfort, 'sitting on a ball', pelvic pressure or back pain. It has a huge impact on the quality of life of individuals and also has an economic impact on the patients and healthcare systems. Risk factors include vaginal births, age. Race menopause, increased intra-abdominal pressure and pelvic surgery including hysterectomy. Assessment of prolapse entails evaluation of bowel, bladder and sexual function. Treatment may take a conservative approach with pelvic floor muscle training before surgery is undertaken. The choice of treatment and route of surgery are individualized to each patient. Post hysterectomy prolapse presents even greater challenges and thorough patient assessment and counselling is essential. The surgeon must have the right skills and choose the right operation to ensure optimal outcome. The surgery itself can be undertaken vaginally or abdominally (open, laparoscopic or robotic), by use of native tissue or mesh and ideally in a multidisciplinary set up.

Keywords: hysterectomy, vault or vault prolapse, recurrent prolapse, surgery for prolapse, mesh for prolapse, quality of life

1. Introduction

Pelvic organ prolapse is defined as the symptomatic downward displacement of pelvic organs usually through the vagina. The incidence is 3–6% based on symptoms but as high as 50% based on examination as a majority of the women are asymptomatic [1].

Risk factors for prolapse include previous vaginal deliveries, assisted/difficult vaginal deliveries, complications after hysterectomy, heavy physical work, neurological disease, hysterectomy for pelvic organ prolapse, and family history of pelvic organ prolapse.

There is no agreed definition of pelvic organ prolapse after hysterectomy. The International Continence Society (ICS) joint report defines it as "descent of the apex of the vagina after hysterectomy" [2]. The route of hysterectomy does not seem to be of consequence in developing prolapse later and subtotal hysterectomy does not prevent development of prolapse. Efforts should be made to support the top of the vagina at the time of hysterectomy. Techniques that have been employed

IntechOpen

include McCall's culdoplasty, attaching the posterior vaginal wall to the uterosacral ligaments and sacrospinous ligament fixation.

The incidence of post hysterectomy vaginal prolapse ranges from 0.2 to 43% [3, 4] according to older case series but more recently the incidence has been quoted at 11.6% if hysterectomy was done for prolapse and 0.2% for non-prolapse benign cases [5]. A large Austrian study revealed the incidence of post hysterectomy prolapse to be between 6 and 8% [6].

2. Relevant clinical anatomy

The pelvic floor comprises skeletal muscle (levator ani and coccygeus), urogenital diaphragm, endopelvic fascia and perineal body. The levator ani comprises of pubococcygeus, ileococcygeus and puborectalis muscles. The striated muscles are under tonic contraction. The pelvic diaphragm provides a hammock which anteriorly has a defect or hiatus that allows passage of urethra, vagina and rectum.

The striated muscles of the pelvis contain both slow and fast twitch fibres. Fast twitch contract suddenly with increased abdominal pressures while slow twitch fibres maintain the muscle tone over a long time.

The perineal membrane or urogenital diaphragm is a dense fibrous tissue which spans the anterior part of the outlet and provides attachment for vagina, urethra and rectum. The perineal body lies between the vagina and anus and provides attachment for pelvic floor muscles.

Uterine support (De Lancey I) comprises of uterosacral and cardinal ligaments which are attached to the cervix and upper vagina. Uterosacral ligaments comprise of smooth muscles and form the medial border of the Pouch of Douglas while cardinal ligaments comprise of connective tissue and pelvic blood vessels. At hysterectomy providing support to these ligaments is key in avoiding vault prolapse regardless of the route of hysterectomy. The round ligament helps maintain anteflexion and version of the uterus whereas the broad ligament is just a fold of peritoneum and both have no role in supporting the uterus.

The middle third of the vagina is attached laterally to the arcus tendineus fascia pelvis, a condensation of obturator and levator fasciae (De Launcey II). Anteriorly this condensation is called pubocervical fascia and posteriolaterally it is attached to endopelvic fascia over pelvic diaphragm and sacrum by fascia of Denonvilliers (vaginal septum), and extends caudally into the into perineal body (De Launcey III) and cranially into peritoneum of the Pouch of Douglas.

3. Assessment

The general approach to patients presenting with prolapse symptoms entails a thorough and comprehensive obstetric and gynaecological history followed by a general, abdominal and pelvic examination. A review of risk factors which can be modified is essential as well as asking direct questions regarding bladder, bowel and sexual function. The impact on the quality of health should be assessed including time off work, relationships and coping mechanisms documented.

Table 1 shows the International Continence Society's POPQ (pelvic organ quantification system) [7] which is used to assess pelvic organ prolapse. It has 6 points which are all measured at maximum Valsalva except total vaginal length. **Table 2** shows the criteria for staging.

Point	Description	Range of values
Aa	Anterior vaginal wall 3 cm proximal to the hymen	−3 cm to +3 cm
Ba	Most distal position of the remaining upper anterior vaginal wall	−3 cm to +tvl
C	Most distal edge of cervix or vaginal cuff scar	−10 cm to +10 cm
D	Posterior fornix (N/A if post hysterectomy)	
Ap	Posterior vaginal wall 3 cm proximal to the hymen	−3 cm to +3 cm
Bp	Most distal position of the remaining upper posterior vaginal wall	−3 cm to +tvl

Table 1.
POPQ system.

Stage 0	Aa, Ap, Ba, Bp = −3 cm and C or D ≤ − (tvl – 2) cm
Stage I	Stage O criteria not met and leading edge < −1 cm
Stage II	Leading edge ≥ −1 but ≤ +1 cm
Stage III	Leading edge > +1 cm but < + (tvl – 2) cm
Stage IV	Leading edge ≥ + (tvl – 2) cm

Table 2.
POPQ staging criteria.

4. Management

4.1 Conservative management

Prevention of prolapse is important and measures should be taken to avoid conditions that increase intra-abdominal pressure. Constipation and chest conditions such as chronic obstructive pulmonary disease (COPD) should be treated adequately. Weight loss is key and hormone replacement therapy may help reduce the incidence. Antenatal exercises, proper intrapartum care and timely caesarean section are also important in reducing the incidence of prolapse.

Initial management should involve appropriate counselling and initiation of pelvic floor muscle training. The best outcomes have been seen when a trained physiotherapist is involved. A perineometer and biofeedback device can be used. Vaginal cones and electrical stimulation have been shown to be effective in incontinence management but no data is available regarding efficacy on urogenital prolapse.

There is a role for devices including vaginal pessaries. They are either silicone or polythene and come in different sizes. They are inserted into the upper vagina and support pelvic organs. They can be cleaned and replaced every 6 months which gives the practitioner a chance to check for any complications. Special attention and counselling should be done with regards to regular changing, sexual function and small possibility of side effects including vaginal discharge, infection and rarely fistula formation.

4.2 Surgical management

The definitive management of post hysterectomy vaginal prolapse is surgery. This should be done by an appropriately qualified surgeon following thorough assessment and counselling of a patient. Different routes of surgery should be considered and discussed with patient. The choice of surgery depends on type of prolapse, age of patient, previous surgery, comorbidities, surgeon's skills and level of sexual and physical activity.

The aim of surgery is to restore normal vaginal anatomy and restore sexual, bowel and bladder functions. In studies, restoration of apical vagina (Point C on POPQ) to 0 or I is used as the measure of prolapse treatment [8].

The type of surgery chosen should be individualised to the patient. This would depend on concomitant prolapse in other compartments, previous prolapse surgery, previous abdominal surgery, sexual activity, presence/absence of bowel or urinary symptoms, total vaginal length, presence of comorbidities and patient's preference.

Abdominal sacrocolpopexy can be undertaken via open or laparoscopic route. Patient selection is vitally important. It is the route of choice for women with a short vaginal length, those who require concomitant abdominal surgery and those with history of dyspareunia. The vaginal vault is fixed to the longitudinal ligament on the anterior part of the sacrum using a permanent mesh. Abdominal sacrocolpopexy is associated with lower rates of recurrence, dyspareunia and post-operative stress urinary incontinence compared to sacrospinous ligament fixation [8]. Common complications include infection, bleeding from presacral veins and mesh erosion. Laparoscopy may not be available in all centres and the learning curve is long.

Robotic sacrocolpopexy is available in limited centres around the world owing to the huge cost associated with setting up.

Sacrospinous ligament fixation entails fixing the vaginal vault to the sacrospinous ligament on one side using absorbable or non-absorbable materials. For right handed surgeons this tends to be fixed to the right sacrospinous ligament. No benefit has been shown for bilateral compared to unilateral fixation. It is associated with low recurrence, high satisfaction and takes a short time to perform and a short recovery time. Common complications include buttock pain, pudendal nerve injury, high recurrence of 8–30% of anterior compartment and ureteral obstruction.

High uterosacral ligament suspension (HUSLS) is also an acceptable procedure for vault prolapse but should not be offered as a first choice and should be undertaken by a well-trained pelvic floor surgeon owing to the risk of complications. An RTC comparing high uterosacral ligament suspension and sacrospinous ligament fixation and found the two similar in terms of anatomical, functional and adverse effects [9]. Complications of high uterosacral ligament suspension include bladder injury, ureteric injury, urinary tract infection, blood transfusion and bowel injury.

Transvaginal mesh involves use of permanent mesh to support the vaginal vault to the uterosacral ligament bilaterally in order to restore level I supports. It has been withdrawn in most centres around the world owing to safety concerns and complications. An RTC compared transvaginal mesh and laparoscopic sacrocolpopexy and found that laparoscopic sacrocolpopexy had longer operating time but better success rate and patient satisfaction at 2 year follow up and women in the transvaginal mesh group had shorter vaginal length and risk of erosion [10].

Colpocleisis is the complete closure of the vagina when sexual activity is no longer desired. It can be used to treat vaginal vault prolapse after hysterectomy following careful assessment and counselling. It has the advantage of being minimally invasive, can be done under regional anaesthesia and the technique is easy to learn. Several techniques are known including purse string closure [11], vaginectomy [12], colpocleisis after performing standard anterior and posterior vaginal wall repair [13], purse-string closure of enterocele followed by approximation of perivesical and rectovaginal fascia and high levator plication [14] and le Forte's colpocleisis [15].

It is recommended that one inserts a mid-urethral tape for cure of stress urinary incontinence at the time of surgery if the vaginal route is chosen. Colposuspension has not been shown to be effective in these patients. In case of recurrent vault prolapse post hysterectomy, the case should ideally be discussed at a multi-disciplinary team before an appropriate plan is made regarding the type of surgery and the person to undertake it.

5. Conclusion

Post hysterectomy vaginal prolapse is a challenging condition that requires adequate evaluation, counselling and appropriate management plan. It is becoming commoner because of increased longevity, withdrawal of vaginal meshes and changing techniques of fixing the vault at hysterectomy. Risk factors should be sought and appropriate measures taken to reduce these. Conservative care should always be attempted when appropriate before surgery. Surgery should be undertaken by a suitably trained surgeon ideally in a multidisciplinary set up.

Author details

Johnstone Shabaya Miheso
Nairobi Urogynaecology Center, Nairobi, Kenya

*Address all correspondence to: jmiheso2001@yahoo.co.uk

References

[1] Barber MD, Maher C. Epidemiology and outcome assessment of pelvic organ prolapse. International Urogynecology Journal. 2013 Nov;**24**(11):1783-1790. DOI: 10.1007/s00192-013-2169-9

[2] Haylen BT, de Ridder D, Freeman RM, Swift SE, Berghmans B, Lee J, et al. International Urogynecological Association; International Continence Society. An International Urogynecological Association (IUGA)/International Continence Society (ICS) joint report on the terminology for female pelvic floor dysfunction. Neurourology and Urodynamics. 2010;**29**:4-20

[3] Symmonds RE, Pratt JH. Vaginal prolapse following hysterectomy. American Journal of Obstetrics and Gynecology. 1960;**79**:899-909

[4] Barrington JW, Edwards G. Posthysterectomy vault prolapse. International Urogynecology Journal and Pelvic Floor Dysfunction. 2000; **11**:241-245

[5] Marchionni M, Bracco GL, Checcucci V, Carabaneanu A, Coccia EM, Mecacci F, et al. True incidence of vaginal vault prolapse. Thirteen years of experience. The Journal of Reproductive Medicine. 1999;**44**:679-684

[6] Aigmueller T, Dungl A, Hinterholzer S, Geiss I, Riss P. An estimation of the frequency of surgery for posthysterectomy vault prolapse. International Urogynecology Journal. 2010;**21**:299-302

[7] Bump RC, Mattiasson A, Bø K, Brubaker LP, DeLancey JO, Klarskov P, et al. The standardization of terminology of female pelvic organ prolapse and pelvic floor dysfunction. American Journal of Obstetrics and Gynecology. 1996;**175**:10-17

[8] Maher C, Feiner B, Baessler K, Schmid C. Surgical management of pelvic organ prolapse in women. Cochrane Database of Systematic Reviews. 2013;**4**:CD004014

[9] Barber MD, Brubaker L, Burgio KL, Richter HE, Nygaard I, Weidner AC, et al. Eunice Kennedy Shriver National Institute of Child Health and Human Development Pelvic Floor Disorders Network. Comparison of 2 transvaginal surgical approaches and perioperative behavioral therapy for apical vaginal prolapse: The OPTIMAL randomized trial. JAMA. 2014;**311**:1023-1034

[10] Maher CF, Feiner B, DeCuyper EM, Nichlos CJ, Hickey KV, O'Rourke P. Laparoscopic sacral colpopexy versus total vaginal mesh for vaginal vault prolapse: a randomized trial. American Journal of Obstetrics and Gynecology. 2011;**204**:360.e1-360.e7

[11] DeLancey JO, Morley GW. Total colpocleisis for vaginal eversion. American Journal of Obstetrics and Gynecology. 1997;**176**:1228-1232; discussion 1232-5

[12] Hoffman MS, Cardosi RJ, Lockhart J, Hall DC, Murphy SJ. Vaginectomy with pelvic herniorrhaphy for prolapse. American Journal of Obstetrics and Gynecology. 2003;**189**:364-370; discussion 370-1

[13] Harmanli OH, Dandolu V, Chatwani AJ, Grody MT. Total colpocleisis for severe pelvic organ prolapse. The Journal of Reproductive Medicine. 2003;**48**:703-706

[14] von Pechmann WS, Mutone M, Fyffe J, Hale DS. Total colpocleisis with high levator plication for the treatment of advanced pelvic organ prolapse. American Journal of Obstetrics and Gynecology. 2003;**189**:121-126. 96

[15] Pelosi MA 3rd, Pelosi MA. Transvaginal needle suspension with LeFort colpocleisis for stress incontinence and advanced uterovaginal prolapse in a high-risk patient. The Journal of the American Association of Gynecologic Laparoscopists. 1998;**5**:207-211